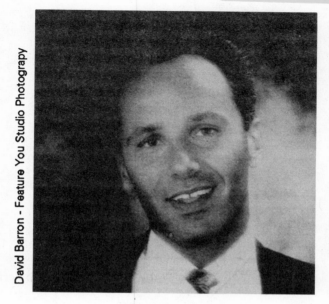

Adam J Jackson is a practising iridologist and physical therapist from London. He runs a private clinic in North London and another in Toronto, Canada. Adam originally trained, qualified and practised Law as a solicitor in England before re-training in natural health therapeutics including Iridology at the International Institute of Iris-diagnosis in Germany. He is a member of the Royal Society for the Promotion of Health, the London and Counties Society of Physiologists, and he is founder president of the Canadian Institute of Iridology.

ALTERNATIVE HEALTH

IRIDOLOGY

A GUIDE TO IRIS ANALYSIS AND PREVENTIVE HEALTH CARE

ADAM J. JACKSON

ILLUSTRATED BY SHAUN WILLIAMS

Charles E. Tuttle Company, Inc.
Boston • Rutland, Vermont • Tokyo

This book is dedicated to the memory of my Mother.

IRIDOLOGY

First published in the United States of America by
Charles E. Tuttle Company, Inc.
of Rutland, Vermont, and Tokyo, Japan, with editorial offices at
77 Central Street, Boston, Massachusetts 02109

ISBN 0-8048-1833-9

Cover art by Isabella Groblewski
Cover design by Fahrenheit

First Printing 1993

Printed in the United States of America

CONTENTS

Part III
Foresight – a preventive health lifeplan

PREFACE

I first became interested in health when, as a child of 14 I was suffering from the so-called 'incurable' skin disease called psoriasis. It was characterised by red scaly blotches that, more often than not, itched so badly they felt as though insects were crawling under my skin.

I remember there was a time when I was so badly affected that I had to be hospitalised for intensive treatment, and it was one day during my stay that an incident occurred that was to change my life. I overheard the doctor speaking to the woman in the room adjacent to mine during his lunchtime rounds. Like myself, she was also suffering from psoriasis, and the doctor noticed that she had not touched a large portion of her lunch, namely the lamb chops. The doctor asked her why she had not eaten all her food, and she told him that every time she ate lamb, or other fatty meats, her skin erupted.

The doctor, who, I might add, was not a lowly house doctor but a top dermatologist, then raised his voice to the woman and told her in no uncertain terms that what she ate could in no way, shape or form affect her skin, and that she should be grateful for what she was given. Even to me, a child of 14, the doctor's words were more difficult to swallow than the hospital food. Something did not seem to make sense. After all, if, as we were taught in biology classes, the food we eat becomes part of us, was it not then obvious that food may affect our skin?

By the end of my hospital stay, and after continuous coal-tar baths and repeated applications of ointment and pastes, and being daily wrapped up in Saran wrap like a half-eaten piece of cucumber, my skin had got better, although still not fully cleared. I asked the nurse if I was now 'cured' and she sat me down and told me as sympathetically as she could that nobody with psoriasis is 'cured'; everybody has to go back to hospital once a year or, if you are lucky, once every other year at the very least.

I was determined not to have to return to hospital. And, thank God, I have never had to. Instead I began my search for the secret of health, something that has taken many years and which still continues. My passion grew, to such an extent that I gave up my position as an attorney and decided to study and work full-time in the field of natural health. My search has brought me into contact with dedicated people who have taught me, inspired me and helped me find my way. And, along the way, I have come across many important truths, but none more so than the one that I set out below and which encapsulates the message of this book.

For every effect there is a cause; for every ailment there is a remedy; for every problem there is a solution; for every event there is a purpose, a reason, and a lesson.

When we ask, we receive; when we seek, we find; when we knock, the door opens.

There is a light at the end of every tunnel. And in the tunnel of ill-health and dis-ease, the light of health is in the eye.

ACKNOWLEDGMENTS

I would like to give special thanks to my dear friend Edith Just B.A.A.R. and her late husband Dr. Emile Just, two extraordinary people who first helped and guided me into the natural health field.

My thanks also to Derek Spivack, optometrist, for giving me the opportunity of working alongside him; to Dr Daryl Irving for his assistance in research of the book; to Perter Cox and Peggy Brusseau for their encouragement when I first considered writing this book; to Peter Roberts of Compassion In World Farming and also to the Jewish Vegetarian and Ecological Society for their help and information; and finally I would like to thank my family and friends (particularly my brother Mark who arranged access to a computer for me so that I could finish typing the manuscript after mine had broken down).

I would also like to thank William Heineman Ltd. and Harcourt Brace Jovanich Inc. for their kind permission to use the extract from *The Little Prince* written by Antoine de Saint-Exupéry.

HOW TO USE
THIS BOOK

This book can be read, like any other, from beginning to end. However it has been designed to be an easy reference guide, enabling you to find out, through self analysis of your eyes, what type of constitution you have (i.e. the condition and character of your body), your major constitutional strengths and weaknesses, and then what dietary and other measures you take to optimise your level of health and avoid disease.

In Part I of the book the fundamentals of iridology and simple techniques of iris analysis are explained in order to enable you to analyze your own irides for a basic understanding of your constitutional weaknesses and strengths.

Part II of the book shows you how to design your own individual preventive health care programme using only natural remedies (including herbal and homoeopathic preparations, and tissue salts). It also gives practical dietary advice, and simple naturopathic treatments that assist the body's own healing force to deal with the underlying causes of disease as recorded in the eye, rather than merely treating symptoms.

Part III explains the general principles of preventive health care, emphasising the importance of diet and nutrition, posture and exercise, and emotional states.

As a final note, if you are taking any medication or are under the care or supervision of your doctor or hospital, or if you have any condition for which you are receiving treatment, you should seek the advice of your doctor before starting any of the remedies outlined in this book.

1
INTRODUCTION

> The true healing art is one in which we teach the patient to change his living habits to conform to natural laws so that instead of having to rebuild a sick body, he can prevent disease in the first place.

> Bernard Jensen, *The Science and Practice of Iridology*

This book is about you. It is about using an age-old technique to look through your eyes deep inside your body and discover the state of your health. It contains the blueprint for building a better and healthier future.

LOOKING AT THE BODY THROUGH THE EYES

Iridology is the science of analysing the iris of the eye. It is a unique form of health analysis – a simple painless non-invasive method of diagnosing your constitutional strengths and weaknesses, and, literally, the condition of each and every organ inside your body. It sounds remarkable, as indeed it is.

My interest in iris analysis was first stimulated many years ago by a very special lady – an acupuncturist and naturopath. I had been very unwell at the time and, as part of the initial consultation, she had looked into my eyes. Her subsequent diagnosis of the state of my health had been uncannily accurate. I was therefore intrigued and fascinated, and decided to read a little around the subject from any books I could find.

Then one day I found myself talking to a lady during an interval at a physical therapy seminar. Whilst we were talking, the light caught her face and I noticed a large black pigment situated just above the position of three o'clock in her right iris. This area in the eye records the condition of the tissue in the lower throat and thyroid gland, and so I asked the lady if she had a problem with an under-active thyroid gland. She looked at me as if I was a magician, but before she could answer I continued, 'Is it the right side of the gland that is affected [the left iris, which shows the left side of the body, was clear] and have you had the condition for some years [the darkness of the discoloration indicated it to be a chronic condition]?

I can still picture the look on her face, which can only be described as one of utter amazement. She replied 'How on earth did you know? I have been on thyroxin for 14 years and it was the right side of the gland that was surgically removed!' To guess such a specific analysis is virtually, if not totally, impossible, so I knew then that I would have to study in much more detail this curious science of iridology.

This book is the result of much of that study, and of my subsequent practice of iris analysis. It is by no means a definitive textbook on iridology, or an in-depth study of natural medicine, nor is it so intended. It is simply designed to give a practical understanding of how your eyes reflect the state of your health, followed up with simple advice on how to reach optimum health by strength ening constitutional weaknesses and stimulating under-functioning organs as recorded in the iris. It is a means to discover who and what you are, and it provides the foundations on which to build the person you can become.

POSITIVE AND PREVENTIVE

When they learn of iris analysis, many people think of it as frightening; they say that if there is something wrong with their health they would prefer not to know about it. But in reality they are not frightened of iridology or what it might reveal: they are frightened with themselves, with their belief in themselves and their ability to change to create a better future. Everyone wants health, but very few people want to do things necessary to create health; too few people are willing to make the effort to change their lifestyle.

Iridology is positive, and it is preventive. Although the irises only show the state of the tissues inside the body, they record changes in the tissue long before clinical symptoms develop. If you knew that you had weak kidneys, would you choose to drink much alcohol? If you knew you had a build up of cholesterol deposits in your arteries, would you choose to eat high-fat foods? And if you knew that your lungs were badly congested or weak, would you choose to smoke? Perhaps you would, in which case this book will be of little interest to you.

However, in my experience most people who find themselves ill with conditions like diabetes, hardening of the arteries, heart disease or kidney failure, usually adhere to the dietary and other guidelines recommended by their doctor or hospital dietician. But doesn't it make more sense to deal with a condition before it becomes a major health problem?

LENGTH AND QUALITY OF LIFE

In Chinese medicine there is an old saying: 'One disease brings long life; no disease brings short life.' This teaches us that those people who know and understand what is wrong with them usually take care of themselves accordingly, and live a long life. However, those people who think that they are perfect usually neglect their weaknesses and ignore or suppress minor symptoms, and as a consequence they live shorter and poorer quality lives.

Iris analysis gives you a better understanding of yourself so that you can improve not just the length, but also the quality, of your life. Some people's immediate response is to say that they would prefer to live five years less and enjoy themselves; smoking 50 cigarettes a day, drinking 5 beers a day, and eating chocolate bars every day makes for their enjoyment in life. However, their thoughts eventually change when they learn in later life that the body does not work in that fashion; bed-ridden with emphysema, forced to inject themselves with insulin three times a day or facing a premature and often painful

3

death with cancer, they soon realise how wrong they were. They realise that quality of life does not depend upon cigarettes, alcohol and chocolate bars, but upon giving and receiving, upon laughter, upon action, and upon finding a purpose and fulfilling a potential.

ONE MAN'S ORANGE IS ANOTHER MAN'S POISON

We are all unique. Each of us has different physical and emotional qualities.

Have you ever wondered why one person can smoke 50 cigarettes a day for 20 years and suffer no noticeable symptoms, whereas another person smokes the same amount for only a few years and develops bronchitis, emphysema, or even cancer? Why is it that one person thrives on emotional stress whereas another has a nervous breakdown? What is it that enables one person to eat cream cakes, chocolates and sweets without putting on any weight, whereas another person only has to look at a dish of ice cream to put on 5 pounds?

It is simply because we are all different, each of us blessed with different strengths and weaknesses. Some people have strong lung tissue whereas others have weak lungs. Some people have fast metabolisms – they convert food into energy very quickly and therefore do not put on weight – whereas others have slow metabolisms and gain pounds in weight whilst eating only moderate amounts of food.

HOW TO SELECT THE BEST NATURAL REMEDY

Many people who feel below par go to a health-food store or drugstore and purchase a selection of vitamin and mineral supplements or try one of the numerous elixirs. However, most times this trial and error game is a complete waste of time and money.

But if they could discover why they were feeling below par, they could select the right remedies. For instance a feeling of chronic fatigue and lethargy may be due to poor nutrition from an imbalanced diet, or it may be the result of poor absorption of nutrients due to excess acidity or toxicity in the digestive tract. It may even be that there is nervous exhaustion or poor blood circulation. The remedy in each case will be different because, to eliminate the problem, we must find, and deal with, the cause of the problem.

THE SEED OR THE SOIL?

Different seeds need different conditions in the soil before they can flourish; it is the condition of the soil that is crucial to the growth of the seed. An apple seed needs lush fertile soil and a temperate climate to grow into a tree and give fruit, whereas a fig tree needs dry sandy soil and a hot climate to grow and produce fruit. It is the soil and the climate that either nourish or eliminate the seed and that determine its growth. And if the soil will not accommodate it, the seed cannot grow.

Similarly, it is the condition of your body and not the virus that determines your state of health. Take a bowl of tomatoes and bruise one, and you will soon see that that is the one that attracts bacteria first. Similarly an organ or area of tissue must be weak or congested to fall prey to a germ or virus.

All viruses and germs are irrelevant in preventive medicine because they cannot survive in a healthy bloodstream. If this were not so, why is it that a particular virus produces a disease in one person but not in another? The germ is not the determining factor in disease; the determining factor is you – your constitution and the state of your immune system, and this can be seen in your eyes.

LOOKING FOR THE CAUSE

Health is not a matter of luck – it is a matter of cause and effect. Nothing happens by chance, and nothing happens overnight, particularly in the matters of health and disease. We were not created to be ill; we were created to be healthy. Health is the natural state of being and the result of living in harmony with the laws of nature.

On the other hand, disease (or dis-ease) is totally unnatural – the result of breaking the basic laws of nature. All disease (dis-ease) has a small beginning; it is a slow insidious process in which a part of the body gradually weakens and becomes congested, creating the right conditions for disease to manifest.

But what if you could discover your constitutional strengths and weaknesses? What if you could see areas of congestion in the body before they manifested themselves as symptoms? What if you were given the opportunity to prevent possible dis-ease? What if ... you could save your life.

THE ROAD TO HEALTH

The eyes are like a road map, showing us the direction we must travel to find health. Seen in this light, iridology is anything but frightening. It is enlightening. What is frightening is to live a live in fear – fear of cancer, fear of heart disease, fear of chronic degenerative disorders, fear of the future. Too many people life with such fear.

This book is about letting go of that fear. It is a book about preventive medicine rather than fast cures. It is about the law of cause and effect. It is about reaching optimum levels of health rather than avoiding disease. It is a book principally designed to enable you, the reader, to take charge, to take control and to take responsibility for your health.

PART I
IRIS ANALYSIS

To know others is wisdom,
To know oneself is enlightenment.

Lao Tsu

The camera lens slowly zoomed in and focused on David Suchet's eyes. Mr Suchet was playing Leopold Bloom in a television production of Joyce's *Ulysses*. Although this particular shot lasted for less than 30 seconds, it was a tense moment in the programme – and one that may well have saved the actor's life.

A doctor who happened to be watching the programme noticed a large arcus senilis or cholesterol ring in Mr Suchet's eyes. An arcus senilis is a whitish ring around the periphery of the iris, and is more commonly found in elderly people, for it indicates hardening of the arteries by cholesterol and mineral deposits. The doctor immediately wrote to Mr Suchet suggesting he had a check up.

'I went to a heart specialist', Mr Suchet explained, 'and tests confirmed a dangerously high cholesterol level which could have led to a fatal stroke. I was so frightened I became like a monk; gave up all the "naughties" foodwise, and restricted myself to fresh fruits, salads, low-fat yoghurt, garlic and lecithin supplements. The result was that my cholesterol level shot down, as did my weight. I have never been in better shape or more full of energy.'

Needless to say Mr Suchet was extremely grateful to the viewing diagnostician. The technique of iris analysis outlined in this book probably saved Mr Suchet's life – it may well save yours.

2
THE LIGHT OF THE BODY

The light of the body is in the eye: when the eye is sound the body is sound.

Matt. 6, 22

During the middle of the last century one man stumbled across a discovery which I believe will yet change the course of medical history. The discovery began with a child playing with an owl in his back garden, and led to what is now referred to as iridology. Throughout the ages the eyes have been proclaimed as the windows to the soul, yet only in relatively recent years has the full truth of this statement begun to be appreciated.

Iridology is the science of analysing the iris (the coloured part of the eye) in order to determine the condition of the organs and tissue of the body. The eyes can be likened to miniature television screens, recording the cellular activity throughout the body. For under magnification they reveal in minute detail the state of the tissues throughout the body – inflammation, toxicity, acidity, degeneration, spasm, lymphatic congestion, hardening of the arteries, the heart, the liver, gall bladder, kidneys, pancreas, spleen, thyroid gland, lungs and bronchials; they are all recorded in the coloured part of the eye known as the iris.

Iridology is by no means a new science; history records that the eyes have been used to diagnose a person's health for literally thousands of years. Hippocrates, the father of medicine, referred to the eyes in his diagnoses, and evidence suggests that numerous groups of people, including the Jesuits, the Brahmins and the monks of Tibet, centuries ago, knew that the colours of the eye were influenced by diseased conditions of the body. It has also been reported that stone slabs found in Asia Minor depicted the iris and its relationship to the other parts of the body.

The principles of iridology have also been known and practised for some time in Europe. *Chiromatic Medica*, published in 1670 and written by Phillippus Meyens of Dresden, mentions iris markings, while a Scottish physician called Keogh Murphy wrote his *Practitioner's Medical Treatments* in 1735, again quite clearly noting the relationship of the eye to the state of health of the patient. Subsequently, however, until the time of the First World War, this idea was considered by the medical profession as preposterous.

THE FOUNDER OF MODERN IRIS ANALYSIS

It is written that 'the prophet shall be considered a fool', and it is certainly true that prophets are rarely recognised for their true worth in their own lifetime. Yet it is their depth of perception and love for humanity that follows them, and those living in later lifetimes who are willing to listen to the echo of the prophet's words receive the blessing. The prophet of this book is a Hungarian medical doctor called Ignatz von Peczely, who was born on 26 January 1826. As with many other universal truths, the eyes as 'windows of the soul' were opened to him as a result of an accident and astute observation.

I was only eleven years old, when one day I tried to catch an owl that defended itself violently, and plunged its claws into my hand, and the more I tried to free my hand the deeper did the owl, with its claws pierce my flesh. There was no other way but to try by force to break the one leg of the owl in order to extract the claw, and as I was a strong boy I succeeded in doing so.

During the struggle I and the owl chanced to look each other sharply into the eyes, and the very moment I broke the leg in two, I observed to my surprise a black streak appearing in one eye of the owl. However, a friend of animals, I took the bird home, bandaged its leg, and treated it until it again was well during which time the bird became so tame that it returned and ate at my table in the garden, and continued doing this a long time after it was liberated.

In the fall of the year the owl flew away, but next summer it returned and was quite tame as it had been the previous year. And one day sitting with it on my hand, I happened to notice the black streak in the one eye of the bird, and saw that it was there just as plainly as on the day when it originated, but it was now bordered and surrounded by white lines!

Extracted from *Iris Science*, Dr H.W. Anderschou (1916).

The boy became a man, and the man a physician. One day when he was consulted by a patient suffering from a broken left leg, the incident with the owl re-entered his memory. Could it possibly be that the patient's eye had changed in the same way as the owl's eye had done? He took a magnifying glass and gazed into the patient's eye. Sure enough, at six o'clock in the left iris, there was a dark streak. Excitedly he examined the eyes of all the patients in the waiting room, and in the months and years that followed discovered an indisputable correlation between the markings of their eyes and his patients' diseases.

In the subsequent years Peczely was able to construct a map of the eye, locating the areas that recorded the various organs of the body, and in 1880 he published the result of his work and investigations in a scientific journal. He then visited England to take part in a medical congress in London, where he gave a lecture on 'Diagnosis through the eye' to a private audience of doctors, but it is recorded that the president of the congress would not allow the lecture to be published as the subject was considered 'absurd'. This was a great disappointment to Peczely, who returned to Budapest somewhat broken. To that disappointment was added the tragic death of his wife and, from that time forth, he gave up fighting for his discovery.

Neils Lilequist, a Swedish pastor during the 19th century, was said to have discovered the changes of colours in the iris independently from Peczely. More recently, many others have worked to bring iris analysis to the attention of a wider public, including: Dr Anderschou of Norway; Australian born Dr Henry Lahn; Dr P. Thiel, Pastor Felke, Dr R. Schnabel and Joseph Deck of Germany; Dr J. Kritzer and Dr Henry Lindlahr of the USA; Dr B. Jensen from the USA, a leader in this field for over 50 years; Dr R. Christopher and Dr D. Bamer, both of the USA; and, more recently, Dr V. Ferrandiz of Spain and Dorothy Hall of Australia.

This book is a small part of that struggle, a faint echo of Peczely's cry, a cry which itself has been heard throughout the ages: 'The light of the body is in the eye'.

3
THE WINDOWS
OF THE SOUL

In ancient cultures the eye was considered the gateway
to the soul, and to the physician today, the eye serves as
a window through which the state of health can be
readily observed.

Patrick D. Trevor Roper, *Lecture Notes in*
Ophthalmology (6th edition)

Your eyes are unique, as individual as your fingerprint –
they are part of what makes you special. Eyes are not just
for seeing; they light up your face and brighten your smile.
The most beautiful woman in the world will not appear
attractive if her eyes are harsh and hateful. Similarly, the
plainest of girls can be the centre of attraction when her
eyes become bright and sparkle.

The eyes are often the first form of communication
between two people, and it is from the eyes that first
impressions are formed. Most of us instinctively analyse
other people with whom we come into contact every day
by the appearance of their eyes – more so, perhaps, than
any other physical appearance or mannerism, because the
eyes reflect moods, character and physical well-being.

One researcher in this field, John Nash Ott, Director of
the Environmental Health and Light Research Institute in
Florida, concluded from his studies and experiments that
different coloured light rays actually create different
emotional states (*Health and Light*, Devin-Adair, USA,
1973). For instance, blue light causes a feeling of well-
being, whereas an orange/pink light causes aggression and
anger. He found that minks, normally fierce creatures,
became docile and friendly when clear windows were

replaced by deep-blue coloured panes. Similarly, baseball players lost their hyper-aggression and irritability when their pink-tinted sunglasses were replaced by a mid-grey tint.

At the same time as our moods are affected by what the eyes see, the eyes also reflect the changes in our moods. It is well known, for instance, that the pupil enlarges when we see someone to whom we are attracted, and when under tension the pupil is reduced in size. And what causes the change in the size of the pupil? The iris.

THE EYE IN NATURE

The workings and effects of the human eye are truly wondrous. When Charles Darwin was asked how the human eye evolved, he replied that even to think that the human eye had evolved would be 'absurdity in the highest degree'. Why? Because the eye is a complete marvel. A perfect video-camera, focusing images, refracting light and recording information better than any photographic equipment we could possibly imagine. Of this Darwin was aware; what he did not know was that the eyes are even more than cameras; they are also like miniature television screens, recording information from inside the body.

A closer investigation of eyes reveals a whole world of untold mysteries. For instance, the chameleon is a reptile renowned for its ability to change colour to camouflage itself within its environment. Although it had been assumed for many years that the cause of the change of colour was the chameleon's fear, this in fact is not so, for a chameleon cannot change colour if its eyes are covered. What is perhaps even more interesting is that if only one eye is covered, the corresponding side of the chameleon's body will not change colour. Similarly, fish that have the power to change colour do not do so if their eyes are covered. The winter hare in Scandinavia can change the colour of its fur from white to brown, but again this change will not occur if its eyes are covered; in fact, there was a report of a winter hare with only one side of its pelt white and the other brown, a closer examination revealing that the animal had one eye missing.

In common with the rest of nature, our eyes affect and reflect our physical bodies. The eyes are the first organs in the body to register minor illnesses such as fatigue and nervous tension, and even cold and flu viruses cause them to become swollen, watery and puffy. But the eyes give the first indications, not only of specific conditions inside the body but also of many so-called 'diseases'.

MODERN MEDICINE AND IRIDOLOGY

Even orthodox medicine now accepts that the eye is an indicator of many health problems, ranging from diabetes to a stroke, from anaemia to goitre. These and other diagnoses are made by examining the condition of the blood vessels of the retina at the back of the eye, by the general appearance of the eyeball and socket, and by looking at the whites of the eyes (sclera). However, the orthodox medical establishment has for the most part completely ignored the relevance of the iris.

True, there are many doctors, particularly in Germany and Australia, and a number in the UK and USA, who use iris analysis but until properly controlled clinical trials are

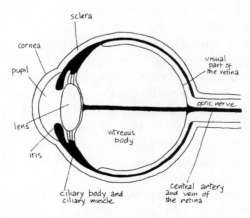

PARTS OF THE EYE

undertaken (which takes a lot of time, a lot of money, and a lot of goodwill and co-operation from a reputable hospital or medical centre to give the trials credence), the medical establishment will continue to ignore the relevance of the iris as a health indicator.

There have been two studies on iridology recorded in the medical literature, one to test for stones in the gall bladder and the other on kidney infection: P. Knipschild, Department of Epidemiology and Health Care Research, University of Limburg, The Netherlands, 'Looking for gall bladder disease in the patient's iris' *British Medical Journal,* December 1988 and A. Simon, D.M. Wosthen and J.A. Mitas, 'An evaluation of Iridology, *JAMA,* September 1979. However both trials were given controls and parameters that were inappropriate for iridology. As regards the first study, virtually every textbook on iridology states quite clearly that gallstones cannot be seen in the iris. The iris only records the condition of the body tissue; gallstones will therefore never show up in the iris, although if their presence is inflaming the surrounding tissues, then the inflammation will become apparent. In the latter study the iris was used to identify kidney infections, but a similar problem occurred here because the iris cannot identify clinical diseases. It can and does record changes in the tissue, and therefore inflammation and excess acidity will be visible. But not all people with excess acidity recorded in the area of the iris relating to the kidney will have a clinically demonstrable 'infection'.

It seems logical that the best method of conducting trials to validate iridology clinically would be to examine the irises of people with broken limbs. This type of test gives acceptable parameters and will result in a straightforward 'Yes' or 'No'. It was, of course, through a broken limb that modern iridology began. However, to carry out such a study requires time, money and the co-operation of a busy hospital fracture clinic.

There may be many reasons why medicine continues to neglect iridology. Modern medicine is mainly concerned with alleviating or suppressing symptoms, whereas the iris reflects causes, not symptoms. For instance there are many possible reasons why a person may suffer a migraine. He may have eye-strain, he may have a vertebra displaced in his neck, or he may have an intolerance to certain foods. Although a tablet may get rid of the migraine, it won't even slightly affect the underlying cause and therefore the patient's irises will not improve. In fact the markings in the irises will more than likely worsen, due to the toxic side-effects of the medication.

Modern medicine is also mostly concerned with pathology or medically-named diseases, whereas the iris does not point to or identify a 'disease' as such. Degenerative diseases including cancer, diabetes and pneumonia are not confirmed in the iris; however toxicity and congestion of lymph tissue, weak tissue in the pancreas, and inflammation of the lungs and bronchials will be apparent. The iris reflects only the state and condition of the body tissue, and from this a remedial treatment programme can be designed to deal with all the body systems rather than treating the 'disease' in isolation.

In fact, treating a 'disease' can often be very misleading, simply because many diseases have similar symptoms. For instance, a sharp pain in the right side of the lower abdomen is often 'colic' (muscular spasm of the intestines) but it may also be appendicitis (inflammation of the appendix). Whilst both are extremely painful, colic is not particularly dangerous, while appendicitis is potentially life threatening. This is in fact the reason why most people who suffer acute pain in the right side of the lower abdomen have their appendix removed, even though after the operations it has been shown that only one in four of them actually have had an inflamed appendix.

Focusing on a so-called 'disease' is also often extremely negative and destructive, particularly where the 'disease' is considered to be incurable. I remember a young lady who had been feeling lethargic and suffering terrible fatigue, and who had been to a hospital for various tests. She was subsequently told that she had multiple sclerosis (MS), a crippling degenerative disease of the nervous system for which there is no known 'cure'. Although she had been fatigued, she had been able to walk into the hospital; but after being told she had MS, she had to be taken out of the hospital in a wheelchair.

Another important difference between the philosophy of modern medicine and that of iridology is that modern medicine considers a person to be healthy if he is not sick. A patient may, for example, have ulcerative colitis and experience pain and bleeding from the rectum. With allopathic medicine the patient is considered well when the pain can be suppressed; the doctor is then considered to have done his job, even though the eyes still show the build-up of acidity and inflammation. Suppressive medications may actually produce a worsening of the underlying condition as demonstrated in the iris. In iris analysis a person is healthy only when the tissue is clear and the elimination channels are functioning.

But perhaps the main reason why orthodox medicine has continued to ignore the iris is that, to date, no one fully understands how, or indeed why, the iris records the condition of the tissue in the body. But how important is it to know how it works? How much do we know of the mysteries of life? We have plenty of labels to describe phenomena – magnetism, gravity, love, electricity – but do we really understand how they work? Do we understand the motion of the waves? Do we understand the life-force? Do we understand how one corn seed left inside an Egyptian pyramid for over 3,000 years still contains within it the ability to germinate when planted? In the words of Socrates, 'The more I know, the more I know I don't know'.

In medicine, in particular, we still know very little. For instance, we don't know why a display of sincere affection speeds up the healing process, in some cases by up to three times. We don't know why, if a needle is placed at a specific point on the skin, the brain releases endorphins and encephalins, nature's way of alleviating pain. But do we need to know how something works before we are willing to use it? If so, then perhaps we should stop holding

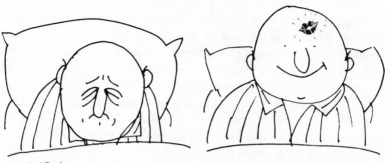

A DISPLAY OF SINCERE AFFECTION SPEEDS UP THE HEALING PROCESS
— BY THREE TIMES IN SOME CASES ....

hands or embracing each other until a scientist or researcher somewhere can understand how a hug can create a feeling of well-being and encourage recovery from illness.

THE IRIS–BRAIN CONNECTION

For whatever reason, the iris is still described by most medical dictionaries, almost derisively, as simply a group of ciliary and concentric muscles which control the amount of light entering the pupil. But whilst this is one function of the iris, there is more to the iris than meets the eye!

The eyes and the brain are closely related. In the embryo the eye starts out as part of the brain. It then slowly separates, yet remains connected to the brain via the optic nerve and optic thalami, and the sympathetic and para-sympathetic nervous systems. The iris is in fact an extension of the brain, being endowed with literally hundreds of thousands of nerve endings, microscopic blood vessels, muscles and connective tissue. And the nerve cells within the iris appear to record the vibratory rate of cells in other parts of the body, and respond to change in body tissue. The markings and colours in the iris change as the condition of the body tissue changes.

The eye, and more particularly the iris, is a very complex organ about which we still know very little. But we do know that there is a terribly intricate connection between the eye and the brain via the nervous system. We do know that the eye and the iris both change in form with changes in our body chemistry.

The different markings, colours, and structural deviations in the iris indicate the state of the tissue in a specific area of the body. Although nobody fully understands how it works, empirical observation confirms that the iris has a reflex action that corresponds to specific changes in the tissues of the body and to the exact location of these tissues.

At first it may seem complicated. After all, if all the organs of the body are recorded in the tiny area of the iris, shouldn't it be an intricate procedure and far too complex for a lay person to comprehend? Not for a basic health analysis it isn't. In actual fact, and as you will shortly discover, it is really quite simple. Let's start by looking in your eyes . . .

4
WHAT TO LOOK FOR IN AN IRIS

God be in my Eyes, And in my looking.
God be in my Mouth, And in my speaking.
God be in my Heart, And in my thinking.

Sarum Missal

Like any science, analysing an iris can be a complex and
very lengthy procedure, especially as the newly developed
video-iriscope incorporates the very latest optical photographic equipment, and provides a totally new system of
analysing an iris at very high levels of magnification.
Today we are able to see things in the eye that have never
been seen before. Research has been put on a new level,
and slowly we are discovering the incredibly minute detail
recorded in the iris, down to such specific conditions as
blocked fallopian tubes.

To illustrate this level of detail, I recall an incident
shortly after opening up a clinic in Mayfair, London. I was
visited by a reporter and photographer from a local news-
paper. They asked if I would analyse their eyes, which of
course I did. The video-recordings took a few minutes to
take and I then went through brief analyses. The
reporter's blue irides had deep, lacunae (holes) in the lung
and bronchial areas, showing weak degenerated tissue. He
then informed me that only a year or so earlier he had had
tuberculosis of the lungs. The photographer's eyes were of
a mixed colouring, and showed digestive disorders. Then,
as we looked at the left iris, I pointed to a lesion which
appeared in the lower abdomen, 'around the tissue of the
left testicle'. He looked at me completely dumbfounded.
'How on earth did you know that? Only last week I had an

operation to remove a growth from my left testicle!'

Of course to analyse a person's condition in that sort of detail takes years of training, study, practice and equipment with high magnification. However, if we stick to the basic conditions and analyse the main body systems, it is not as complicated as you might at first imagine. And the same rule applies for remedial and preventive treatments; if we tackle the main conditions and keep the elimination channels open, the body will take care of the smaller conditions.

In this chapter, therefore, I have set out a simplified and structured approach to analysing an iris. In a general iris analysis there are four basic steps involved:

- What is the base iris colour?
- What is the general iris structure?
- What is the general iris constitution?
- What is the condition of the main body systems and elimination channels in the body?

However, before starting to analyse an iris, it is necessary to become familiar with iris topography via the iris charts. We must know where the various organs and systems of the body are recorded in the iris.

THE IRIS CHART

The iris charts have evolved over the last 100 years. The greatest strides in this area were, of course, made by Peczely, but modern advances in optical photography have enabled much more detailed charts to be developed. Although iris charts produced by different schools of iridology may show slight discrepancies, these discrepancies relate to minor detail and all the charts remain fundamentally the same.

The chart I have developed through my practice may look complicated at first, but there is an easy method of memorising it. The first thing to notice is how the right iris records the organs on the right side of the body, and

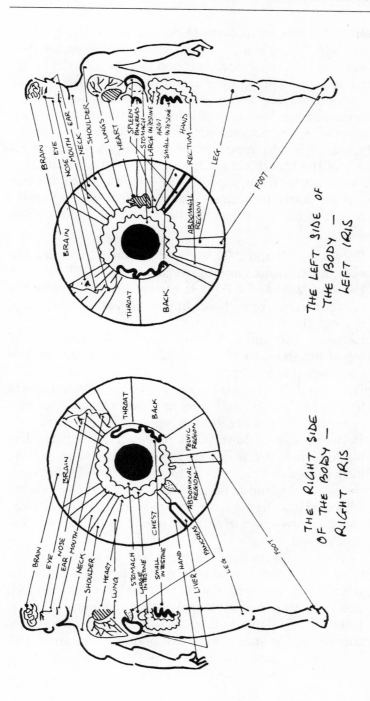

THE LEFT SIDE OF THE BODY — LEFT IRIS

THE RIGHT SIDE OF THE BODY — RIGHT IRIS

similarly the left iris records those organs on the left side of the body. There is a sound physiological reason for this: the optic nerves cross sides between the eye and the brain, which is why, when someone suffers a stroke, it will appear in the opposite eye to the side of the brain in which the haemorrhage has occurred; however the nerve connections cross again between the brain and the rest of the body, which is why a stroke on the left side of the brain will affect the functioning of the right side of the body.

If we start with the right iris and look at it as a clock face, it all starts to become clear – see how the various parts of the body are located between the hours on the clock?

- Between 1.00 and 2.00 is the upper face, including the eyes, nose, sinuses and upper jaw.
- Between 2.00 and 3.00 is the lower face, including the lower throat, bronchus, upper throat, mouth and thyroid gland.
- Between 3.00 and 4.00 is the upper-back region – the top of the shoulder blades to midway down the back to the lower thoracic spine.
- Between 4.00 and 5.00 is the lower-back region where the lower thoracic and lumbar vertebrae, sacrum and coccyx (tailbone) are located.
- Between 5.00 and 6.00 is the pelvic region. The bladder lies immediately next to the sacrum, the kidney lies in this area between 5.30 and 6.00, and the adrenal gland is immediately on top of the kidney. The rectum, penis and prostate in men, and the uterus and vagina in women, are of course all in this area as well.
- Between 6.00 and 7.00 is the lower abdomen. In this region we have the appendix on the right side, the peritoneum (muscular wall in the abdominal cavity), and the ovary in women and testicles in men.
- Between 7.00 and 8.00 is the upper abdomen, containing the major digestive organs – the liver, gall bladder and pancreas.

12 RADIAL SECTIONS

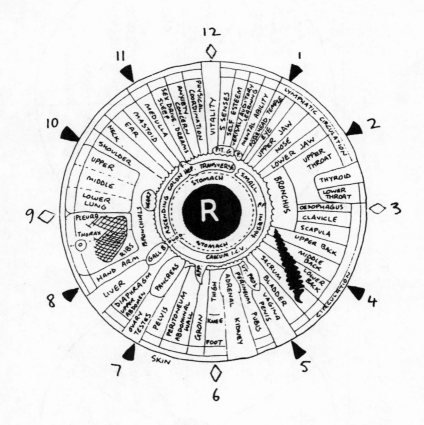

THE IRIS MAP – RIGHT EYE
(looking at another person's right eye)

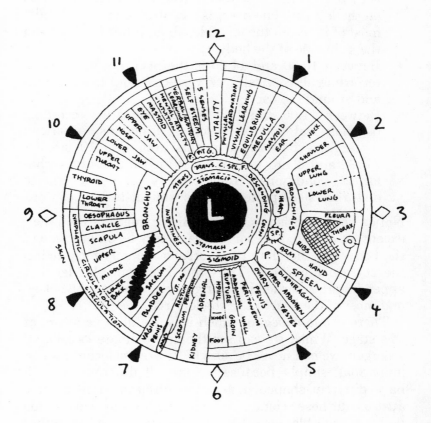

THE IRIS MAP – LEFT EYE
(looking at another person's left eye)

- Between 8.00 and 9.00 is the chest and breast area, recording the ribcage and breast.
- Between 9.00 and 10.00 is the lung and bronchials, with part of the heart being recorded here, as well as on the left iris. The heart is a central organ and, whilst most of it lies on the left side, about a third of it lies on the right side of the body.
- Between 10.00 and 11.00 is the neck and ear region, recording all cervical neck vertebrae and the tissue in and around the ear.
- Between 11.00 and 1.00 is the head area, recording psychological and physiological functions. American researchers have divided this area into 10 smaller zones, and claim to have identified different psychological conditions, from anxiety and concern to disturbed sleep patterns and sexual disturbances.

Notice how one iris is simply a mirror image of the other, except, of course, that some organs only lie on one side of the body and therefore those organs are only recorded in the corresponding iris. Thus the liver, gall bladder and appendix are recorded in the right iris, whereas the spleen and most of the heart lie in the left iris.

There is one *caveat* of which it is useful to be aware at this stage. Whilst we can see the approximate location of an organ, we can never be sure of its precise location in an individual, simply because we are all different. We all have different-shaped bodies and different-sized organs. Just as our noses come in various shapes and sizes, so too do livers, gall bladders, kidneys, hearts, and all the other internal organs; for example, some people have larger livers than others, and some people have larger spleens than others. The area of the iris covered by an organ will therefore depend upon the organ's size.

THE CIRCULAR ZONES IN THE IRIS

The radial division of the iris in the form of a clock face as explained above shows the location of affected tissue. But once we establish the location of a potential or existing problem, we then need to find out which tissue in the area has been affected. We may, for instance, find a marking in the left iris between 7 and 8 o'clock, which relates to the left side of the lower back; but is it a trapped nerve, a muscular adhesion or a displaced vertebra?

The different tissues and body systems are recorded in circular concentric rings going around the iris, from the pupiliary edge to the outer edge of the iris.

- Stomach.
- Intestines.
- Veins, blood.
- Muscle.
- Skeletal.
- Lymph.
- Arteries, blood.
- Skin.

Again there is an easy way to remember this division, by dividing the iris into three equal sections.

- The innermost section contains the organs of preparation and absorption, i.e. the stomach, which prepares and breaks down the nutrients ready for absorption through the small intestines. Although the

THE CIRCULAR ZONES

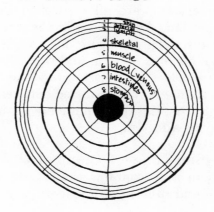

large intestine eliminates body wastes, it has been claimed that some nutrients, most notably vitamin B12, are manufactured in the large intestine and absorbed through its wall.

- The median section contains the organs of utilisation, and includes the pancreas, gall bladder, heart, adrenal and pituitary glands, the autonomic nervous system and the blood and lymph vessels in and around the abdomen. Falling within this zone are also the muscles, tendons, ligaments and bones.

- The outer section contains the main organs of detoxification and elimination, detoxification occurring through the liver, spleen, kidneys, lymph and lungs, and direct elimination occurring through the nose, mouth, urethra, anus, and, of course, the skin itself.

The Inner Zone – Organs of Absorption

The innermost zone of the iris relates to the stomach, and immediately next to that lies the intestines. The wreath going around the pupil is known as the autonomic nerve wreath (ANW) and is a convenient landmark distinguishing the intestines from the venous blood zone next to it.

The ANW shows not only the shape and condition of the intestines, but also the state of the autonomic nervous system. The autonomic nervous system controls all major body functions that you cannot consciously or directly affect; for example your heart beat, your digestion, your hormonal system, are all controlled by the autonomic nervous system. Any breaks in the wreath or discolourations or distortions indicate an adverse condition of the autonomic nervous system, and will affect the part of the body to which the distortion in the iris relates. For instance, if the ANW is distorted between 9 and 10 o'clock in the right iris, the right chambers of the bronchials and lungs may be affected.

The Median Zone – Organs of Utilisation

The median zone contains the organs and systems that distribute and utilise the nutrients. The first zone in this section is the blood zone, relating primarily to the venous blood flow. It is in this zone that the signs of varicose veins first appear. Toxins in the system and the build up of acidity in the blood will also be indicated in this zone.

The muscle tissue lies next to the blood zone and records changes in all the soft tissue – muscles, tendons and ligaments. However it is sometimes not easy to distinguish the muscle zone from the skeletal zone, as they lie next to each other with little to differentiate them. A joint condition will always affect the soft tissue around it because the surrounding fibres become strained; likewise, a condition affecting the soft tissues will in a short time affect the joint itself because it is only the soft tissues that hold the joint in its correct position. If tissues on one side of a joint become injured and weak, the joint will be pulled out of its correct alignment by the stronger tissues on the other side.

The Outer Zone – Organs of Elimination
The outer zone of the iris contains the main detoxification and elimination channels – the skin, lungs, liver, rectum and the penis/vagina. The concentric rings within it represent the lymphatic system and the arterial system, while on the very outer edge of the iris is the skin zone, showing up any problems with the skin itself.

IRIS COLOUR

There are many different colours of iris, ranging from brown to hazel, grey to blue, but they can all be divided into three main categories of base colours – blue, brown and mixed.

Blue and brown were originally thought to be the only pure base colours of iris, and any deviation between blue and brown therefore represented a chemical change in the body which may have been inherited or acquired. Indeed the change of colour in the iris was first observed in the last century by a Swedish pastor called Niels Lilequist, who noticed how his own blue eyes became green after he had been given large doses of quinine to deal with a malaria infection.

Today, with the prevalence of inter-marriage among the races, there are many base iris colours. However, there is no ideal colour, in much the same way as there is no ideal iris; each has its own strengths and weaknesses. What is certain is that the iris should be a uniform and clear colour, whether blue/grey or hazel/brown. A clear iris indicates healthy functioning of all the major elimination channels in the body. Once congestion sets in and the function of an organ becomes affected, the colour in the iris will change in the area relating to the affected part of the body.

The proliferation of chemical pollution in water, food and the air is perhaps another reason why pure iris colours are becoming increasingly rare.

The Blue Iris

The blue/grey iris base colour is found in Nordic, European and Anglo-Saxon races and indicates that the person has a constitution that is more prone to 'acid' conditions such as arthritic, rheumatic, asthmatic and ulcerative ailments. They generally have thinner blood and a tendency to cold extremities, lymphatic congestion and weak kidneys.

The Brown Iris

The brown iris base colour, on the other hand, is found only in Asian, African, Native American and Semitic races. It shows thicker blood and a tendency to digestive disorders, including biliousness, gastricatony, constipation and auto-toxicity, and dysfunction of the nervous system.

The Mixed Iris

A mixed iris is one that is a mixture between blue and brown, more often than not appearing green/hazel. There are of course many variations between the two colours of blue and brown, but it is possible to arrive at a convenient classification. Many times we see a mixed iris that is a green/hazel colour, sometimes with brown colouring around the pupil and extending outwards; to the naked eye this can appear brown, but it is distinguishable from a true brown iris by the fact that the latter has a 'sandy' texture throughout, whereas a blue or mixed base colour iris has clearly defined fibres radiating from the pupil to the periphery of the iris.

The mixed colour iris has a genetic blue base, and makes the person susceptible to acid and toxic conditions. This person needs to take special care of his/her body (particularly the digestive and nervous systems) by regular cleansing and good living habits in order to maintain a sound level of health and avoid dis-ease.

DISCOLOURATIONS IN THE IRIS

On top of the base colour we often find other colours dotted around the iris and these reveal the 'functioning' of the tissue or organ, whether hyper (over-active) or hypo (under-active), acutely inflamed or chronically congested, loaded with toxic waste or even degenerating. These 'top' colours point to abnormal functioning of the various body systems.

White
White is the first stage in the dis-ease process, indicating acidity, over-activity and inflammation. It is the acute stage of the condition, and often the person will not be aware of any symptoms when the discolouration first starts to show in the eye. But the area will turn whiter and brighter as the inflammation increases, and symptoms will follow.

Yellow
Yellow is the sub-acute stage of the dis-ease process, indicating the development of acid deposits and toxic congestion within the tissues. This occurs after the acute phase, and indicates a more chronic condition.

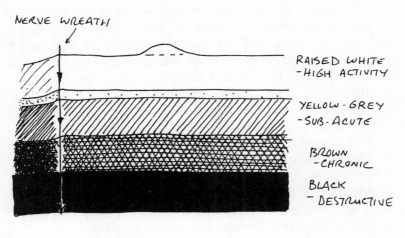

NERVE WREATH

RAISED WHITE
-HIGH ACTIVITY

YELLOW·GREY
-SUB·ACUTE

BROWN
-CHRONIC

BLACK
- DESTRUCTIVE

IRIS COLOUR

A good example is the effect of the common cold. The respiratory tract becomes inflamed, producing mucus to protect the membrane in the acute stage. If typical decongestants are taken, the mucus is dried up rather than being eliminated, and it slowly continues to irritate the membranes and provide a convenient base on which bacteria can breed. Toxicity then begins to accumulate. This, then, is the yellow phase.

Orange/Brown
Orange/brown is the sub-chronic stage, indicating more deep-seated congestion and toxicity. The tissue is now malfunctioning and unable to cleanse itself efficiently, so the person will require a cleansing programme involving herbal remedies to assist and stimulate the body's elimination channels in clearing away the accumulated waste.

Black
Black is the chronic stage, the final and degenerative phase of the dis-ease process, indicating hypo-function and loss of substance of the tissue. It rarely occurs over-

night, except in the case of traumatic injury such as a broken limb.

In this chronic state the body will require further investigation by your health practitioner and a long-term naturopathic course of treatment.

Red

Red discolourations in an iris usually indicate a build-up of iron in an area, which may be caused by taking iron supplements. These are often poorly absorbed by the body and appear to deposit in and around certain tissues in the body. However, internal bruising or bleeding also shows up as a red discolouration in the iris, particularly in the area next to the pupil which relates to the intestinal tract.

Psora

Finally, watch out for the fly in the ointment. There are some discolourations that lie above the iris structure itself. These are known as psora and, whilst they indicate weakness and congestion in the tissue, they are more inherent weaknesses than acquired areas of congestion. This means that it could take a long time for these to disappear from the eye. Don't worry about them; simply take care of the related area.

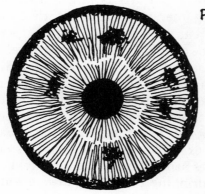

PSORA
PIGMENTATION

THE IRIS STRUCTURE

Iris structure refers to the appearance of the fibres in the iris that radiate outwards from the pupil, and which show the strength of the connective tissue throughout the body.

The body has four basic types of tissue – epithelial tissue (meaning skin or membrane) muscle tissue, nerve tissue, and, finally, connective tissue (meaning everything else). Connective tissue, very simply, is the blood, bone and tissue that connects everything together. The founder of osteopathy, Andrew Taylor Still, said that 'It is to the connective tissue that we must look to discover the cause of disease'. And in iris analysis we do exactly that.

It is the connective tissue that determines and reflects the state of the other body-tissue in the body. This is why the iris does not record stones in the kidney or gall bladder, or natural events such as pregnancy. For the condition of the connective tissue around the kidneys or gall bladder may remain unaffected by stones within those organs, and there is no change in the condition of the tissues during pregnancy unless there are other complications.

In basic terms, the closer the iris fibres are together, the stronger is the connective tissue of the body; conversely, the further apart the iris fibres become, the weaker the tissue. Thus, with one glance we can immediately see our own physiological strengths and weaknesses.

Whilst the structure of the iris is largely determined congenitally and during infancy, parts of the iris structure may be acquired, and can change according to a person's lifestyle, particularly in childhood and adolescence, when tissue is still being formed. It is therefore vital that a child's first seven years are as conducive to building as strong a foundation as possible because it is upon that foundation that the rest of the child's life is supported.

However, structures can be strengthened or weakened by our lifestyles. For example, heavy prolonged smoking may result in the fibres separating in the lung area in the iris, and continuous drinking of alcohol may eventually cause the fibres in the kidney area to tear apart. It really is all a question of cause and effect. What our parents do and we do determines what type of person we will become.

THE FOUR BASE STRUCTURAL TYPES

Whilst all irides are unique, they can be broadly identified and classified into four basic structural types according to the fibre patterns. Most iridologists use cloth/material weave as analogous classifications – silk, linen, hessian and net – the structural strength of each cloth being likened to the physical strength of the body, silk being the strongest and net the weakest.

However, the structure also reflects the person's general personality make-up. For instance, in terms of a person's physical make-up, the silk iris is strongest, but at the same time, the silk person tends towards a hyper-nervous activity and is often easily transformed into a weaker and more excitable emotional state. This is not to say that someone with silk irises has or will suffer nervous conditions or become neurotic or a nervous wreck; this will depend upon what else is happening in the person's business, social and family life. The structure of the iris simply points to a person's general physical and emotional strengths and weaknesses.

However, like the different base colours of the iris, we can see that as far as structure is concerned there is no 'ideal' iris. We all have different strengths and abilities, as well as weaknesses and faults. In Taoist philosophy one is taught to follow one's own inner nature – to keep within one's limits. It is only when we try to put square pegs into round holes that difficulties emerge. We all know how strong or weak we are; we all know our limitations if we listen to our bodies. Yet how many of us do listen, and how many of us continue to try to put square pegs into round holes? Looking at the iris base structure confirms much of what we already know about ourselves but were perhaps afraid to ask.

The Silk Iris

The silk iris has tightly-woven fibres and is the strongest physical structural type, often with efficient metabolism, high adrenal stimulus and good mineral balance. This type of person often has superior energy levels, with the minimum need for rest or relaxation. In fact silk people often find it difficult to relax or sit still, and are always on the go. The tight connective tissue shows physical strength, but if not kept mobile and active the already tight tissue can lead to rigidity of the joints and tension of the organs, which may in turn lead to conditions such as osteo-arthritis, rheumatism and constipation.

Although physically strong, the silk-type person tends towards adrenal hyper-function and overactivity of the nervous system. They usually have strong willpower and straight-lined thinking and can cope with high physical, mental and intellectual workloads. However they get worried and uptight very easily, and over-anxious about trivial things.

Because silk-type people have such strong constitutions they often live with and ignore minor pains and symptoms and, at times, go beyond their limits without dealing with the minor ailments or symptoms until a health crisis occurs. It is this person who can break the laws of nature – smoking, drinking, eating junk food. In the short term they show no adverse symptoms, due to the strong tissue in the body capable of optimum assimilation of nutrients and elimination of waste. But in the long term, toxicity and congestion builds up and degeneration sets in. Any illness therefore tends to be brought on by emotional disturbance, accidental damage, or a prolonged and imbalanced lifestyle.

The Linen Iris

The linen-type iris has looser and more wavy fibres than the silk iris, although with few, if any, large holes or gaps between the iris fibres. The linen structure is the average structural type and the majority of people fall into this category. It reveals a more vulnerable structure than the

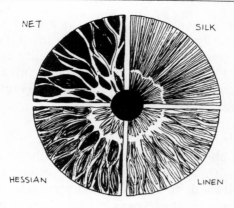

NET   SILK

HESSIAN   LINEN

IRIS STRUCTURES

silk, with less nervous energy, adrenal flow or general physical hardiness. On the other hand, people with a linen structural type also tend to be less physically and emotionally rigid and they have a greater sensitivity to their own and other peoples' needs and physical limitations.

The Hessian Iris

The hessian iris structure contains looser fibres than the linen type, with some large holes in the tissue. This type is below average in structural strength and therefore encounters more health problems if the body is abused physically through poor diet, lack of exercise, etc. Metabolism is slower, due to weaker connective tissue, and this will be more pronounced where the loosely woven connective tissue is in the thyroid area.

It is particularly important for the hessian type person to have a good balanced diet as the body will not be able to throw off waste products or recuperate as fast as the silk or linen types. It is also advisable for this person to exercise to strengthen the tissues, and so avoid underfunctioning of organs, sluggish bowels and poor venous blood circulation (all conditions common in hessian and net structures), augmented and/or caused by flaccid, weak tissue.

On the positive side, the hessian is a person who can relax more easily than the silk and linen types. The hessian-type person tends towards flexibility rather than the rigidity of the silk-type person, both physically and emotionally, and is therefore not as easily affected by emotional stresses.

The Net Iris

The net iris shows large cavities, resembling a spider's web, and is the weakest of the physical structures, tending, if allowed, to low physical strength and under-function. However, these people can often filter out the stresses in their lives and have good energy and health levels, provided, as with the hessian-type structure, they do not physically abuse their bodies through poor nutrition and lack of exercise. If they do fall ill, their powers of recovery and recuperation are slower than those of the other iris types. It is therefore particularly important for the net-type person to prevent physical illness rather than continually to seek cures, because they do not recuperate very speedily. A bout of flu that would cause a sick person to take a day off sick from work might cause a net-type person to take a week or more off to convalesce.

SPOTTING THE WEAK AREAS

Once we have looked for the base structure of the iris we can begin to look at the specific structural markings. A person may have a silk-type base structure but with a large hole in one particular area. Similarly another person may have a net base iris but with one or two areas of very tight connective tissue. Remember, when we look for the structural markings in specific areas of the iris we are looking at the structural strengths and weaknesses of the specific organs – the closer the fibres in the iris, the stronger the related organ. Where fibres start to separate, the related organ is weaker – the deeper the separation, the weaker the organ.

Lacunae

There are many different types of lacunae (holes). However, for basic analysis, all we are concerned about is their location, depth and whether they are 'open' or 'closed', i.e. whether the outer end of it is open or whether it has all sides closed. The importance between this differentiation is that the closed lucana shows the related organ to be in a much weaker condition – the tissue is no longer able to absorb nutrients fully. In the case of the open lacuna, whilst indicating weak tissue, the related organ is still receiving adequate nutrients. Therefore where we see a closed lacuna, more care and a greater effort must be taken to strengthen the tissue and to avoid putting it under undue stress. For example, if we see weak tissue in the kidney area of the iris, it would not be advisable to drink alcohol too frequently or eat a lot of high-protein foods on a regular basis.

Raised Fibres

Raised fibres indicate irritation and often, where the fibres are inside a lacuna, an infection, or damaged tissue resulting from an infection. They are commonly found in the musculoskeletal zones, and point to rheumatic and arthritic conditions in the tissues, the severity of which depends upon the colour of the raised fibres.

Transverse Fibres

Fibres that run diagonally across other fibres are called transverse fibres, and show a fibrosis or scarring in the

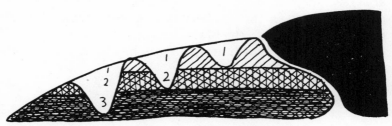

THE LACUNA AND THE LAYERS OF THE IRIS

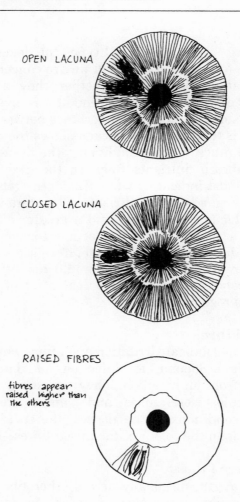

OPEN LACUNA

CLOSED LACUNA

RAISED FIBRES

fibres appear
raised higher than
the others

area (see diagram on p. 52). Whilst it is true that operations rarely show up in the iris because the anaesthesia blocks the nerve response to the brain, it is not uncommon to find a transverse fibre where deep surgery has been undergone.

5
TAKING A GOOD LOOK

When an organ or part of the body undergoes acute or chronic changes as a result of hereditary influences, systemic or drug poisoning, or from mechanical injury, then these pathological changes are recorded in the corresponding area of the iris.

Henry Lindlahr, *Iris Diagnosis and Other Diagnostic Methods*

Specific signs in the iris indicate specific conditions within the body. Set out below are illustrations and brief explanations of the more common iris signs and how they reflect the main body systems. Once the specific conditions in the body are established it is possible to seek out the likely causes for those conditions; once the cause is identified, it can be removed. This is the basis on which to build a preventive health care programme, which we will cover in Part II of the book.

THE DIGESTIVE SYSTEM

The Stomach and Intestines
- Central toxaemia. This is a toxic environment in the stomach and intestines revealed by an orange/brown ring around the pupil, the darker the colour, the more chronic and deep seated the toxicity. This condition prohibits efficient digestion as the toxic environment means that foods cannot be efficiently digested, and often lethargy will result from the inability to absorb or utilise nutrients fully. It can be caused not only by a

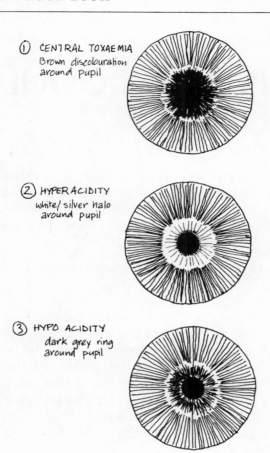

① CENTRAL TOXAEMIA
Brown discolouration
around pupil

② HYPERACIDITY
white/silver halo
around pupil

③ HYPO ACIDITY
dark grey ring
around pupil

junk-food diet that may contain or produce toxins in the body, but also by the long-term use of medications (particularly antibiotics); many medications kill off the protective flora in the stomach and intestines, thus allowing a toxic environment to develop. Negative emotions, particularly anger and depression, also hinder the digestive process and are often instrumental in creating this condition. Whenever central toxaemia is seen, the person's liver will be under stress, for it is the liver's job to filter accumulated toxins from the body, which in this case will have built up in the stomach and intestines.

- Hyper-acidity. A silverish/white ring immediately around the pupil is called an acid ring or acid halo, and indicates excess acid in the alimentary tract caused by too many acid-forming foods and/or emotional stress. The more acid present, the whiter the ring becomes, until the chronic stage, when it becomes grey and later brown. When brown discolouration sets in the acid has, over the period of time, created a toxic environment.

- Hypo-acidity. This is an insufficiency of acids in the stomach, often caused by enzyme deficiency. It is recognised by a grey discolouration in the stomach zone, which generally succeeds the hyper-acidic stage. In this case it is difficult for the intestines to absorb acid-forming foods and a simple diet is required, with optimum food combinations, in order to put as little stress as possible on the digestive process in the stomach.

- Spastic colon. A spastic colon (large intestine) is not as ominous as it sounds. It simply means that the colon wall has lost its tone and is mis-shapen, thus causing erratic bowel movements. It is easily identified in the iris by the shape of the autonomic nerve wreath in the iris, which, in an ideal state, should resemble a complete circle about one-third of the distance between the pupil and the outer edge of the iris. Where the ANW is distorted, with some of it lying close to the pupil and some of it much farther away, the person has a spastic colon, very often accompanied by erratic bowels. A spastic colon usually builds up over a period of many years and is mostly caused by a diet consisting mainly of refined white flour products (e.g. white bread, cakes, biscuits), meats and white sugar foods, all of which are deficient in the adequate amounts of roughage necessary to maintain the peri-staltic (muscular) movement of the colon wall. That having been said, chronic emotional tensions may also result in a spastic colon. When under stress, many people report that sections of their abdomens feel as if they are being squeezed – 'knotting up'. The emotional tension produces physical tension in and around the colon wall that slowly distorts the shape of the colon and its function.

- Tight colon. This is tension in the tissue in the colon wall, causing the colon to squeeze and narrow the diameter of the tube through which the faeces move resulting in constipation. This problem is evident when the ANW is lying right next to the pupil rather than being a third of the distance towards the outer edge of the iris. It generally results from intense emotional stress, particularly in those people who have weaker digestive systems, although, again, a diet containing highly spiced and refined foods may also contribute to this condition.

- A ballooned colon. Where the ANW is stretched towards the outer edge of the iris it indicates that the large intestine is 'ballooned' having lost much of its tone and strength. As a consequence bowel movements tend to be sluggish and the hormonal glands which are recorded immediately outside the ANW in the iris are often affected as a result.

- Impactions. Impactions are old faecal matter stuck to the inner wall of the intestines, and usually arise out of sluggish movements in the bowels. They are identified by black/dark brown holes or pockets inside the ANW. In the colon excess fluid is re-absorbed through the colon walls, and the faeces are then pressed by the peristaltic movement of the colon wall into stools. However, where the faeces move through the colon too slowly, whether it be caused by a diet lacking in fibre or by emotional tension, too much fluid is re-absorbed through the colon wall and, as a result, the faeces become sticky and hard and cling to the colon wall, resulting in putrefication and fermentation. This will also create a reflex effect in other parts of the body, depending upon the location of the impaction, e.g. if there is an impaction in the ascending colon it may create a reaction in the liver, breast or lung; in such a case, even if symptoms are suffered in areas other than the colon, remedial treatment should commence with cleansing the bowels.

It is interesting to note that, embryologically, the intestines are the first tissues to be formed, after the brain and eyes, and it is from the intestinal tissues that most of the other body organs and tissues are formed. This may be one reason why there is such an intimate connection between the intestinal tract and the rest of the body.

The Main Digestive Organs

- The liver. This is the largest gland in the body and has over 500 known functions. It is therefore not surprising that when the liver is under-functioning the body will suffer in various ways, including a build up of toxicity within the tissues, particularly in the stomach and intestines. In the iris the liver lies between 7.45 and 8.00 in the right eye. All toxicity in the body will be due to an under-functioning liver, as it is the liver's job to filter toxins. Such under-functioning may be caused by: a diet high in fats, sugars, alcohol, and artificial chemical flavourings, colourings and preservatives; drugs and medications, all of which have to be broken down by the liver (even those applied externally, such as hydro-cortisones used in ointments for skin conditions); and emotions of anger and frustration.
- Gall bladder. The gall bladder is recorded in the iris diagonally above the liver and next to the duodenum, into which it secretes bile to help break down fats. Its principal task is to store bile – the main substance involved in the digestion of fats. Foods high in saturated fats (meats, hard cheeses, chocolates, cream, etc.) put additional strain on the gall bladder, and cause gallstones, as well as contributing to a build up of cholesterol within the body.
- Pancreas. The pancreas is located in both the right and left irises, which makes sense as it is a centrally located organ. It has two particularly important functions in the digestive process: the secretion of

pancreatic juices to break down proteins; and the secretion of insulin to control the blood-sugar level. Therefore an under-functioning pancreas will be put under strain if one has a diet high in refined sugars and/or protein-rich foods.

THE CARDIO-VASCULAR SYSTEM

- Scurf rim. This is a darkening around the periphery of the iris indicating poor arterial circulation, particularly to the extremities, which in turn leads to cold hands and feet. It also represents poor elimination through the skin, and is often associated with dermatitis, eczema, psoriasis, acne and other skin complaints.
- Arcus senilis. A whitish or yellowish arc around the upper rim of the iris, indicating poor blood supply to the head caused by hardening of the arteries with cholesterol and/or mineral deposits. This will, if unchecked, lead to hardening of the arteries throughout the body; the arc is then seen completely around the iris and is referred to as a cholesterol ring. This can be a serious condition and it is always worth getting a blood test for cholesterol levels – remember David Suchet (see page 7). Such a condition is generally caused by a diet rich in fats, especially meats and dairy foods. Furthermore, the calcium in cow's milk and cheeses is not efficiently absorbed or utilised by the body, and , taken in excess, it is deposited in the walls of the arteries.
- Weak tissue (heart). A lacuna in the heart zone of the iris indicates weak tissue, although it does not mean that there are, or will be, serious heart conditions. The heart is simply a hollow muscular organ and, like any other muscle, if it is not exercised, atrophy will set in. Weak tissue indicates that the heart is more prone to certain cardio-vascular conditions, which may ensue if the heart is not looked after through diet or exercise, too much stress, etc. It is always those weak areas within the body that experience trouble first: strong

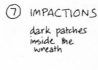

⑦ IMPACTIONS

dark patches
inside the
wreath

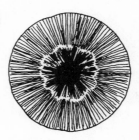

⑧ SCURF RIM

dark ring
around outside
of iris ..

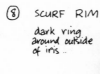

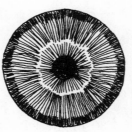

⑨ ARCUS SENILIS/
CHOLESTEROL
RING

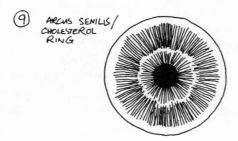

tissue can cope more easily with stress and throw off toxins and infections more efficiently.

THE LYMPHATIC SYSTEM

- Congested lymph node(s). A congested lymph node is seen by a cloud in the lymphatic zone of the iris, and may be acute or chronic, according to the colour of the cloud (white being acute, and brown being chronic). The location of the congested node in the body will, of course, be related to the location of the cloud in the

49

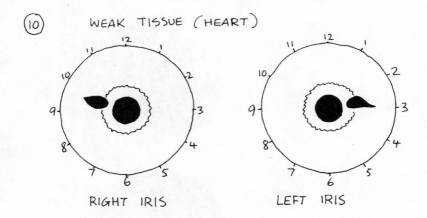

WEAK TISSUE (HEART)

RIGHT IRIS

LEFT IRIS

iris; thus, if the cloud is seen in the left iris between 1 and 2 o'clock, the lymph is congested in the left-hand side of the neck. One man had exactly this sign, a dark cloud at 1.30 in the left iris. However he was totally unaware of any problem and had had no symptoms until he later visited a health spa. Like all the other clients, he was given a range of therapeutic cleansing treatments, and it was immediately after a neck and shoulder massage that the left side of his neck began to swell up to the size of a lemon. The clinic physician advised that the lymph node was chronically congested and the swelling would go down within a few days.

- Rosary. A lymphatic rosary is a circular ring of these white or yellow clouds going around the iris, and points to congestion in the lymphatic system as a whole. The lymphatic system is similar to the vascular system, in that it consists of vessels through which the lymph travels. The lymph nourishes injured parts of the body and collects the waste created by cellular activity. When there is congestion the waste is not eliminated efficiently, making the person more prone to infections, and particularly to allergies, hay fever, swollen glands, etc. In order to overcome the symptoms, the lymphatic system needs to be stimulated and cleansed.

THE MUSCULO-SKELETAL SYSTEM

- Inflammation. Inflamed muscles, ligaments and tendons are seen as a bright white discolouration in the muscular/skeletal zone. This is usually caused by physical injury or trauma, but it may also result from a build up of acid in the tissue caused by eating a lot of high acid-forming foods. If the colour turns darker, the condition is becoming more chronic – usually the case where, for instance, someone with a bad back has taken painkillers over a long period of time. Pain is nature's way of telling us to stop and take remedial action; it is the muscles, tendons and ligaments that hold the joints in place, and if we ignore or deaden the pain, the cause of the back condition worsens, the muscles strain further and slowly pull the joint out of its correct position. What began as a simple muscular strain may then become a chronic and debilitating joint disorder.

- Loose tissue. The presence of lacunae in the muscular/ skeletal zone indicates inherent weakness in the connective tissue in the affected part of the body – areas where one tends to develop the long-standing aches and pains. If there is loose connective tissue in the lower back, that will be the site of injury or discomfort if the person's posture and physical exercise are neglected. Loose tissue is often caused by daily habits that create a poor posture – slouching in front of the television, sitting all day with the phone clasped between the neck and shoulder, always carrying a briefcase in the same hand, always sitting with the same leg on top of the other, and so on.

- Transverse fibres. Transverse fibres are fibres that run across other fibres rather than radiating diagonally outwards, and they indicate distorted tissue and possible deep fibrosis (scarring) or infection in the area in which they are seen. These can be caused by a physical injury or deep surgery, and they may even be congenital.

THE NERVOUS SYSTEM

- Tension rings. Tension rings are circular rings going through the iris, usually found in the muscular/ skeletal zone. They indicate an accumulation of tension and a predisposition to worry and anxiety. Irises containing more than one or two tension rings reveal that the person holds emotions inside and often has a tendency to overreact to stressful situations. If this number of rings is seen in an iris the chances are the person would already know that he or she has accumulated stresses and strains; most people in the modern world have to deal with some sort of stress, but where there are in excess of three tension rings in the iris, the stress is not being dealt with very well. It is often a much needed warning that now is the time to change.
- Tight pupil. A small pupil is a tight pupil. It will usually become small in brightly lit rooms or when a bright light is shone on the eye, in order to restrict the amount of light entering the eyeball and so protect the retina at the back of the eye. However in normal lighting conditions a small pupil indicates that the person is going through, or has recently been through, a period of stress and that the mind and body are only coping by a determined effort. We all do this at times, holding on when deadlines have to be met and

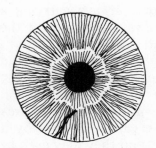

(15) TRANSVERSE FIBRES

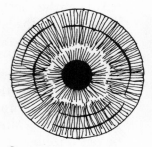

(16) TENSION RINGS

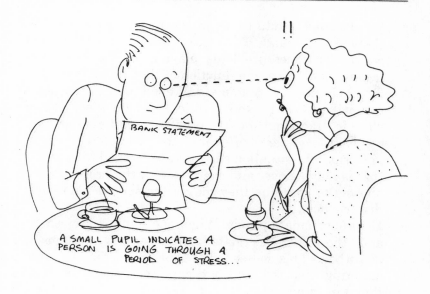

A SMALL PUPIL INDICATES A PERSON IS GOING THROUGH A PERIOD OF STRESS...

promises have to be kept. But in such a case it is better to unwind slowly and plan a break before the stress leads to nervous exhaustion; no one can keep going at a frantic pace or under intense pressure for ever, and it is people who do not listen to their bodies, and who try to keep going without a let-up in the pace, who end up in a health crisis or who collapse from nervous exhaustion.

- Large pupil. A large dilated pupil normally occurs in dimly lit rooms, allowing extra light to enter the eye in order to create a clearer image of whatever is being viewed. However, if a large dilated pupil is seen in normal lighting conditions, it indicates nervous depletion or exhaustion, and usually occurs after a prolonged period of stress, when the pupil was small, as mentioned above. The person in this situation will find it difficult to cope with further stress unless remedial action is taken. Lethargy sets in and the only way people feel they can cope is by taking stimulants in the form of coffee, tea, alcohol and refined sugar foods.

- Head acute. White flares in the head area of the iris (between 11 and 1 o'clock) indicate that recent worries/anxieties/problems playing on the mind are beginning to affect the function of the nervous system.
- Head chronic. A complete darkened area in the head region between 11 and 1 o'clock in the irises shows chronic emotional/mental problems that remain un-resolved and are affecting the person's thought patterns. The situation can often be likened to a record that is playing over and over again; if the problems are allowed to continue they may bring serious emotional disturbance.
- Disproportionate pupils. When one pupil is very small and the other is dilated, the nervous system is disturbed. This is seen in people immediately after suffering a stroke, and it occurs spontaneously. It is therefore advisable, even if no symptoms have been experienced, to have a full medical check to ensure that a haemorrhage from a blood vessel has not occurred in the head.

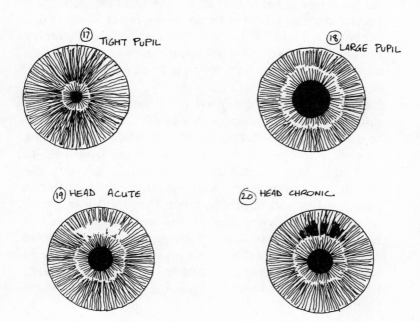

⑰ TIGHT PUPIL   ⑱ LARGE PUPIL

⑲ HEAD ACUTE   ⑳ HEAD CHRONIC

Autonomic Nerve Wreath (ANW)

The ANW is the wreath that runs about a third of the way between the pupil and the outer edge of the iris. It shows the state of the autonomic nervous system (the nervous system controlling all the bodily functions that can be carried out without our conscious control, e.g. breathing, digestion, etc.)

- Inflamed ANW. Where the ANW is inflamed (i.e. bright white) the nervous system has been irritated, either through emotional conflicts and/or a poor diet. Refined foods and coffee, tea and alcohol all deplete the body of vitamin B complex, which is food for the nervous system.
- Orange/brown ANW. If an inflamed ANW is allowed to continue, for instance, when a person is taking artificial nerve stimulants, it slowly turns orange and brown as the condition deteriorates.
- Broken ANW. Where the ANW is broken there will be little or no nerve supply to the related area in the body, with consequent under-functioning of the related

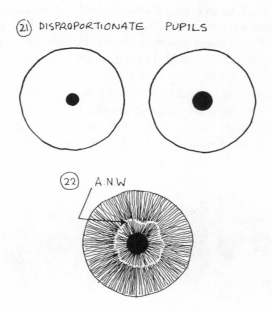

㉑ DISPROPORTIONATE PUPILS

㉒ A.N.W

organ. In this situation remedial measures are necessary to help the body compensate for the damaged nerve. Orthodox medicine teaches that once a nerve is dead, it is dead and cannot be resurrected; however the body can and does compensate for any loss, and new nerve paths may be formed. Where a broken ANW is seen it is advisable to seek a physical therapist to check out the structural condition of the body and also to ensure that the bowels are moving well, as these are two main causes of restrictions in the nerve supply to an area of the body.

THE RESPIRATORY SYSTEM

- Weak/strong tissue. Weak or strong tissue is determined by the fibres in the iris, and is mostly inherited or formed in infant years. This is the reason why one person can smoke for years without apparent symptoms and another person will quickly suffer lung problems. However tissues can and are weakened by lifestyle, whether it be smoking, which affects the lungs and upper respiratory tract, or drinking large amounts of alcohol, which weakens the kidneys and liver. Where there is weak tissue the related part of the body should be well looked after and not abused. Therefore where one has weaker tissue in the lungs, one should do regular exercise, occasional inhalations and avoid mucus-forming foods, in order to prevent unnecessary congestion and to maintain healthy tissue. And of course, not smoking goes without saying.

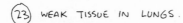

(23) WEAK TISSUE IN LUNGS.

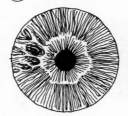
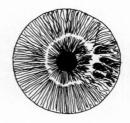

- Congestion. Congestion in the lungs, bronchials, throat or sinuses may be acute (white clouds) or chronic (yellow to brown discolouration). All congestion is caused by inefficient elimination, and is therefore created by eating mucus-forming foods (e.g. dairy foods, sugars, wheat, etc.), smoking and lack of exercise.

THE URINARY SYSTEM

- Congestion in the kidneys. The kidneys lie between 5.30 and 6.00 in the right iris and between 6.00 and 6.30 in the left iris. Congestion again may be acute or chronic, and is seen by the discolouration. Acid deposits build up in the kidneys and can form stones and irritate the membrane. Many people have high acid-forming diets (see dietary guidelines on page 251) and also drink too much fluid; the kidneys filter the blood, and are not flushed by drinking more impure water or other drinks – to drink more fluid when the kidneys are congested is like trying to dance on a broken leg. The kidneys are also referred to in Chinese medicine as the 'seat of the emotions' and are affected particularly by anxiety and concern. If these emotions are prevalent, any unresolved conflicts must be remedied because one can eat the best food in the world and still create acids.
- Congestion in lower urinary tract and bladder. Unlike congestion in the kidneys themselves, a build-up of deposits in the bladder and lower urinary tract leads to cystitis (inflammation of the bladder) and indicates that the urinary tract needs to be flushed, but this must be carried out with due regard to the state of the kidneys, and using herbal support.

THE HORMONAL SYSTEM

The hormonal or endocrine system is an intricate and precise mechanism controlling all the body functions.

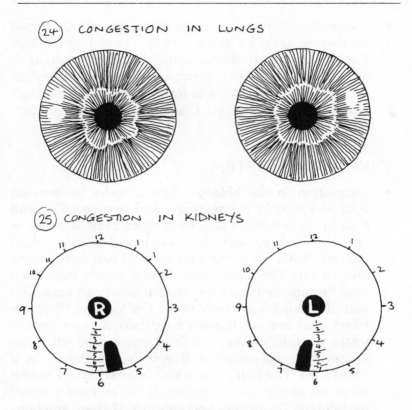

Small and exact amounts of hormones act as catalysts, stimulating specific organs in the body to function properly. Furthermore, hormones are secreted by the various endocrine glands not only in specific amounts but also at very specific times. The functioning of the main endocrine glands can be seen by the strength of the tissue and the colour of the relevant part of the iris.

In this general analysis we will cover only the main hormonal glands.

- The pituitary gland. The pituitary gland is located at 12.15 in the right iris and 11.45 in the left iris, and is known as the master gland as it controls the entire hormonal system. It is this gland that gives instructions to all the other hormonal glands as to when and how much of each hormone should be secreted. Often

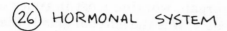 (26) HORMONAL SYSTEM

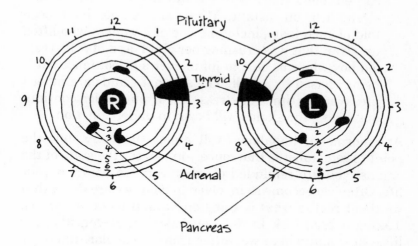

when there appears to be a problem with a hormonal gland, it can in fact be traced back to the pituitary gland.

- The thyroid gland. The thyroid gland, situated between 2.15 and 3.00 in the right iris and between 9.00 and 9.45 in the left iris, controls the metabolism of the body (i.e. it determines the speed at which food is converted into energy). If the thyroid gland under-functions the food is converted very slowly into energy; consequently calories are not burned easily by the body and the person will gain weight. The opposite applies, of course, if the thyroid gland is over-active. However, always bear in mind that the tissue in the iris changes before the physical symptom occurs. If you can see the condition of the tissue, you can take preventive action (this we will cover in Part II of the book).

- The adrenal glands. The adrenal glands lie just above the kidneys in the iris, and are responsible for the secretion of adrenaline – the hormone required in times of stress to make the body work harder and faster. It is the fight or flight organ, working most in times of stress, fear and anxiety; it is the adrenal glands that can enable a small frail woman to have superhuman strength in an instant. Miraculous stories have been told of such feats, including one of a woman who lifted up a van that was crushing her child, and of a 10-year-old boy who was able to jump over a 6-foot fence when being chased by a bull. The adrenal glands are indeed lifesavers in times of stress, but if put under continuous stress, the glands will begin to under-function.

Any hormonal imbalance will affect the body, but the point to remember is that, once you can see the state of the organs, you are reminded of what you are doing in your life. Often we become so involved in what we are doing that we don't realise what is going on around us or within us. Taking a brief look in the eye makes us re-consider our lifestyles, and where we suffer from particular, minor or relatively major symptoms, we can locate the source of the problem from the eye.

6
REFLEX SIGNS IN THE EYES

There is but one remedy for disease; namely, remove the causes that are impairing health.

Dr Herbert M. Shelton

The iris does not indicate symptoms; we cannot, for instance, say whether or not a person suffers migraine or stomach pains simply by looking at an iris. However, by looking into the eyes, we can see past the symptoms and begin to discover the likely causes for the health problems that we may experience.

Symptoms lie outside the realm of iris analysis for several reasons. To begin with, the symptom always appears last in the dis-ease process, and disappears first in the healing process. However, the exact point at which this occurs is not visible in the iris; pain is created, not just by physical pressures or abnormal body chemistry, but also by the individual's ability to feel pain. A small muscle strain may cause great discomfort to one person and yet be virtually unnoticeable to another person. The same physical conditions result in the same tissue changes in the iris, but cause different symptoms and degrees of symptoms.

Furthermore, in any health problem there will be two causes – the underlying cause and the explosive cause. The underlying cause is the weakness or congestion, and the explosive cause is the event that triggers off the pain or symptom. For instance, many office workers frequently hold the telephone between their left shoulder and ear. Over a period of time the neck muscles on the left side of the neck become stronger and the muscles on the right side of the neck become proportionately weaker. Then one day the person turns around or reaches up for something and, suddenly, boom – the person finds himself suffering from acute neck pain, and requires medication and treatment. The act of turning around or reaching up didn't cause the neck problems; it merely triggered off the symptoms, which would not have occurred had not the muscles on the neck already been out of balance.

Similarly, a person may eat a lot of highly acid-forming foods, building up the acid levels in his or her body, until one day he or she is put under intense stress at work and within a day or two experiences severe stomach pains. The stress is the explosive cause, which could not have resulted in such pain had not there already been hyper-acidity in the stomach and intestines. Therefore, if we see hyper-acidity in the stomach and intestines section of the iris, we are not necessarily expecting to see pain; what we are seeing is a tendency to acid problems which, if triggered by an explosive overload of more acid-forming foods or emotional stress, will lead to the related symptoms of pain, ulcers, irritable bowels, etc.

Another reason why the iris does not detect symptoms is that the point of pain is not necessarily the source of the problem or of dis-ease. After all, if a person experiences burning sensations around the heart, it is more than likely being caused by gaseous pressure coming from an over-acidic environment in the stomach. A sharp shooting pain down a leg is often caused by a restricted sciatic nerve in the lower back. Furthermore a specific symptom may have a variety of causes. A migraine may be caused by eye strain, by a crook in the neck, by a food intolerance, an over-burdened gall bladder, or a hundred and one other maladies. The pain is merely the result of what is referred to as a reflex – a foreseeable and involuntary result to a specific stimulus.

WHAT IS A REFLEX?

I remember a lecturer once trying to explain the concept of a reflex to a class of students.

Imagine you are on a safari in Africa, photographing animals. Picture yourself so engrossed in the beauty of the scenery that suddenly, and without warning, you find yourself separated from the rest of the party. You turn around, and to your horror you see a lion standing only yards behind you, looking hungry and ready to pounce. What would be the best thing to do?

One student suggested running away. 'But the lion would be on top of you before you moved a few feet away,' replied the lecturer. Another student said he would climb up the nearest tree. 'Lions can climb trees too, and in any event the lion would have got you long before you could get anywhere close to the nearest tree' countered the lecturer. One by one all suggestions were dismissed, until one student had the courage to ask the lecturer what he would do.

'Well, I would bend down and pick up some excrement by my feet and throw it at the lion. The creature would be so shocked that he would run away', the lecturer said. 'But how do you know that there would be excrement by your feet?' the inquisitive student asked. 'Oh, there would be', countered the lecturer, 'because that is a reflex!'

Most people have experienced how a doctor causes a reflex when, whilst having the patient sit with one knee on top of the other, the doctor slightly knocks a point below a patient's kneecap and the lower leg shoots upward. But there are many other reflexes in the body where a specific stimulus in one part will cause a reaction in another part, far too many to discuss in a book of this nature. However there are some important reflexes of which one should be aware, particularly when analysing an iris.

The reflexes detailed below are particularly useful in pointing to a cause for a symptom from which a person is suffering and for which there is no major disturbance in the related part of the iris. If, for instance, an individual is suffering from violent migraines, there will very rarely be major markings in the head area of the iris, but once you are aware of the main body reflexes you will know where to look for the cause of the problem.

THE THREE IRIS REFLEXES

The Stomach and Intestines

There is an old saying that when everything going into the mouth is pure and clean, and everything coming out the other end is coming out regularly and cleanly, then everything in the middle will be healthy; and there is more than a grain of truth in this.

The stomach and intestines have an intimate relationship with the rest of the body, a relationship that can be traced right back to the embryo. In the embryonic development, the stomach and intestines are the first tissues formed after the brain and the eyes, and it is from the tissues of the stomach and intestines that virtually all of the body's other organs and tissues are formed. It is perhaps for this reason that many conditions all over the body can often be caused by a disturbance in a particular section of the stomach and intestines, the exact location of the reflex depending on the location of the condition in the stomach and intestines. For example, a disturbance in the ascending colon (in the right side of the iris, between 8.00 and 9.00) may affect the right breast, whereas a disturbance in the descending colon (in the left iris between 1.00 and 2.00) may affect the left side of the neck and the left ear.

A good example of this sort of reflex was exhibited by the youngest child of a colleague of mine, who was born with a cyst on the right side of his neck. The child could not be operated on until after his first birthday, and following the operation an x-ray was taken to ensure that everything that should have been removed had in fact been removed. However the picture revealed something totally unexpected; because the child was so small, the area of the X-ray extended down from his neck to his abdomen, and at the bottom of the picture the radiologist noticed an unusual grey area. This revelation prompted a further examination and exploratory surgery, in which it was discovered that the child had been born with a small congenital deformity in the abdomen; a piece of jawbone was lodged in the right side of his intestines, in exactly the location indicated by iris analysis.

Naturopaths and hygienists have for centuries been arguing that many dis-eases and dis-orders in the body can be traced back to disturbances in the intestines. Dr Robert Gray and Dr Bernard Jensen both developed colon cleansing programmes to treat many dis-eases, from breast cancer to epilepsy, with apparent great success. Indeed the whole field of colon irrigation is founded upon this theory.

Adjacent Reflexes in the Iris

It is very common that one part of the body may suffer from a disturbance of its neighbouring tissue or organ. Back pain, for instance, is often caused not by muscular strain in the back but from kidney infection or constipation. When a part of the body is damaged or injured, the surrounding tissue goes into spasm to protect the injured organ, and this may result in pain or symptoms of one sort or another affecting the neighbouring tissues.

Therefore when looking in an iris it is important to consider how adjacent organs may be affecting one another. A numbness around the eyes may be caused by a nerve restriction in the upper jaw, and a pain in the leg, as we have said earlier, may result from a damaged nerve in the lower back. Inflammation in the sacro-iliac section of the lower back may cause bladder disturbances; likewise, weak tissue in the lower throat may affect the functioning of the thyroid gland. However, in iris analysis we are not just considering physically adjacent organs (i.e. those that lie next to each other anatomically in the body), but also those organs that are neighbours by virtue of being located next to each other in the iris. While it is true that very often neighbouring organs in the body are also neighbours in the iris, there are occasions where two organs are recorded next to each other in the iris but are not physically adjacent to each other in the body.

The leg, for instance, does not lie next to the kidney or adrenal gland in the body, but they are adjacent in the iris, and perhaps for very good reasons, for the kidneys affect the muscle and nerve tissue in the lower back, which in turn affect the legs. This is particularly important where remedial treatment is required; a person who suffers a weak bladder and is having to get up throughout the night may have a perfectly healthy bladder that is malfunctioning due to pressure from the sacrum bone in the lower back. In such a case, remedial treatment would be a physical therapy involving remedial massage and/or manipulation. If there was something inherently wrong with the bladder itself, herbal remedies and dietary guidelines, in some cases coupled with reflexology or acupuncture, would be a more appropriate form of treatment.

Therefore when analysing an iris, and before deciding on a preventive health care programme or any form of remedial treatment, it is important to be aware that a disturbance recorded in one area of the iris can cause a reflex disturbance in the organ lying next to it in the iris.

Diagonal Reflexes

In much the same way that parts of the body may be affected by reflexes from other parts of the body represented as lying adjacent to them in the iris, so they may also be influenced by a reflex from those parts of the body situated diagonally opposite in the iris. For instance, pain in the lower back may, in fact, have resulted from an arthritic neck, or a stubborn throat cough may have been caused by congestion in the lungs. Once again, there are often sound anatomical and physiological connections between the diagonal reflexes, as seen in these two examples.

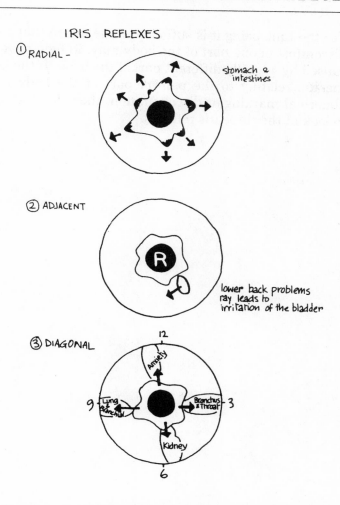

IRIS REFLEXES

① RADIAL -

stomach & intestines

② ADJACENT

lower back problems ray leads to irritation of the bladder

③ DIAGONAL

12

Anxiety

9 Lung and bronchial

Bronchus & Throat 3

Kidney

6

Other diagonal reflexes, such as the connection between anxiety and the adrenal gland and kidney, may not be as obvious, but if we move outside the realms of physical connections in the body and explore the workings of the mind, the relationships often become apparent. And by adding the Chinese perspective to the overall picture, the jigsaw starts to take shape; indeed, the connections independently discovered by iridologists have in fact been known for thousands of years.

These areas we shall explore in subsequent chapters.

For the time being it is sufficient to be aware that pain or discomfort in one part of the body may, in fact, have been caused by a totally different part of the body. If the area in the iris relating to the painful part of the body has no abnormal marking or discolouration, then the next step is to look at the three iris reflexes.

7
THE MIND'S EYE

The mind–body relationship cannot be separated

Dr Bernard Jensen

The human mind is something about which very little is known, even by the foremost researchers in the field of human psychology, and it is extremely doubtful if we shall ever be able to comprehend its magnitude fully. However, through the eyes we are given a glimpse of the state of a person's mind, for the iris does not merely reflect physical health, it reveals a variety of emotional states as well. Stories of anxiety, depression, anger, hypertension, grief and many other emotional disturbances are all told by the eyes.

THE PUPIL

The pupil is nothing more than a small circular black hole in the middle of the iris through which rays of light enter the eye, to be received at the back of the eyeball by the retina.

The amount of light entering the eye is dependent upon the size and shape of the pupils which in turn are controlled by the contraction of the iris fibres. Too much light irritates and may even irreparably burn the retina; but if there is not enough light, the eye cannot see. It is for this reason that, in a brightly lit room, the iris fibres contract radially to reduce the size of the pupil and thereby restrict the amount of light entering the eye; whereas in a darkened environment the iris fibres contract concentrically to enlarge the size of the pupil and therefore allow more light to enter the eye.

The size and shape of the pupil can also be seen as the

size and shape of the iris; they are two sides of the same coin. And for this reason the pupil responds to stimuli other than just different intensities of light, for it is just as surely influenced by a person's emotions and nervous system. It has long been recognized that the pupil reflects the state of the nervous system; for instance, when a person suffers a stroke (a haemorrhage of a blood vessel in the brain), one of the first indications is that one pupil becomes disproportionately enlarged. If the haemorrhage has been on the left side of the brain then the right pupil enlarges, and vice versa.

It is also well known that the pupil reacts to certain emotional stimuli. A good example is that of two people, meeting face to face, who find themselves physically attracted to each other. They become temporarily 'weak at the knees' and both pupils dilate, showing a depletion of nervous energy.

Therefore, after taking into account the influence of light conditions, the pupil size and shape will reflect the state of the nervous system at that moment.

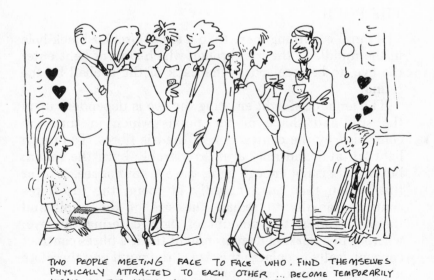

TWO PEOPLE MEETING FACE TO FACE WHO, FIND THEMSELVES PHYSICALLY ATTRACTED TO EACH OTHER ... BECOME TEMPORARILY WEAK AT THE KNEES AND BOTH PUPILS DILATE, SHOWING A DEPLETION OF NERVOUS ENERGY...

The Small Pupil

A small pupil reflects anxiety, tension and nervous strain. It is commonly found amongst people who are going through stressful periods – students prior to examinations, for example, and executives during crucial meetings. But whilst it indicates tension, it also shows a dogged determination to overcome the situation.

Such a person needs to be able to cope with the existing period of stress by taking time to relax, slow down and generally recharge his or her batteries.

The Enlarged Pupil

When both irises are enlarged in normal light conditions, it indicates the nervous system is depleted of energy, such circumstances usually being accompanied by feelings of fear, despondency or despair. Such a situation often follows a period of intense stress; at first the pupil is small, but then, after a time, the nervous system can no longer cope with the pressures and both pupils dilate. A good analogy is that of the physical tension created by a person working out in a gym; for a time the muscles are tense and tighten, straining to lift the weights, but if they continue to lift weights, there will come a time when the muscles feel like jelly – they become too tired to work any further, and collapse.

It is not uncommon for some people suffering with nervous exhaustion to keep 'lifting' themselves by using nerve and energy stimulants such as coffee, tea, sugared sweets and pep-up drinks. But if the person is near to collapsing from nervous exhaustion, the taking of stimulants will only worsen the state of the nervous system in the long run.

The body needs to recuperate and regain its strength, and it needs the right conditions in which to do it. With or without our co-operation, the body will do what it must to rejuvenate; either we take the time to recover, or the body will force us to do just that by bringing on a health crisis.

The Oval Pupil

The healthy pupil is round in shape, and any distortion indicates a more deep-seated condition affecting the emotions. The oval-shaped pupil is a sign of severe psychological disturbance, and some form of counselling and/or psychotherapy is necessary. Early German iridologists went as far as to suggest that an oval-shaped pupil was an indication that the person was suffering from suicidal tendencies.

It is not often that one comes across oval-shaped pupils. In my practices I have only come across a handful. In my first year of practice I was visited by a man whose pupils were vertically oval in shape. He also had silk connective-tissue iris structure. He had been told by his doctor that he was a diabetic, yet, as far as his irises were concerned, there was nothing untoward with his pancreas that could result in diabetes. It transpired that he was taking tablets to control his condition rather than having to inject insulin, even though, as the consultation progressed, it became abundantly clear that there was very little wrong with his pancreas. He had suffered numerous emotional traumas though, most of which he had not been able to overcome; he had deep resentments and regrets, which had culminated in extreme anxiety. In fact his condition was so bad that his doctor had actually forbidden him to record his blood sugar levels for fear he would suffer an anxiety attack.

Whilst most of us suffer various sorrows and hurts in our lives, it is when we allow anger, resentment and other negative emotions to fester that they produce toxins, often more poisonous than any bacterial, viral, chemical or physiological disease. People who have chronic emotional problems need more than just dietary guidelines and herbal remedies; herbal relaxants and calmatives such as valerian root, scullcap, lady's slipper and chamomile are useful, as are Bach flower remedies. Acupressure and acupuncture treatments can produce miraculous results as well. However, most of all, people with deep emotional problems need counselling and some form of psychotherapy.

TENSION RINGS

As we have already mentioned, tension rings (also called stress rings, contraction rings and nerve rings) are visible concentric rings going around the iris, indicating a build-up of tension within the body and a tendency to overreact to what otherwise would be considered to be small irritations – arriving a few minutes late for an appointment, for example, or a minor disagreement. The greater the number of rings, the greater the tension.

Most people these days have one or two tension rings in their irises due to the additional stresses of modern day living, but when more than three rings are visible, emotional tension needs to be examined.

When a tissue in the body tenses, the functioning of the organs around or within it is hindered, blood and lymph flow is restricted and dis-ease follows. Tension rings are mostly found in the medial and outer zones of the iris, their exact location radially and concentrically in the iris identifying the part of the body that is affected by the stress. For example, where the tension rings are concentrated in the muscular and skeletal zones there will be a tendency towards arthritic and rheumatic conditions as the joints start to sieze up and the tissue tightens. If the rings appear in the blood, lymph and skin zones of the iris the tension is more likely to lead to high blood pressure, infections (due to restricted lymph drainage) and skin complaints.

THE AUTONOMIC NERVE WREATH

The autonomic nerve wreath (ANW), as its name suggests, reflects the condition of the autonomic nervous system, and is also affected by emotional strains and stresses. For example, when it has a bright white flare going up into the head region, it indicates a mind full of recent worries that remain unresolved. The darker and wreath becomes in that area, the more long-standing are the troubles and the more irritated is the autonomic nervous system.

THE SOMO-PSYCHOTIC (BODY–MIND) REFLEX

Just as the mind affects the body, so too does the body affect the mind; the various body organs and different parts of the body structure are all affected by specific emotions.

The lower back, for instance, is affected by a lack of emotional or financial support, whereas a frozen shoulder is affected by mental burdens; in fact, it has been considered that as much as 75 per cent of all frozen shoulders are primarily caused by emotional stress. Therefore, when a disturbance is seen in the iris, it may reflect not just the physical condition but also the emergence of a related emotion.

8
THE CHINESE VIEW

Western medicine divides the human anatomy into categories and regards each diseased or malfunctioning part as separate from the whole. In the Orient we believe you are built in one piece, that it is impossible to isolate a part without considering what effect it will have on the whole. We do not concentrate on the illness, but on the entire body. We do not label disease, because all diseases come from the same source – an imbalance of energy flow throughout the body.

Naboru Muramato

For thousands of years Chinese medical philosophy has proffered the view that the mind and body are inextricably linked. As a result Oriental healthcare principles provide interesting and important insights into matters of health, which are particularly relevant to holistic iris analysis. The Chinese approach to health offers not only another means of understanding an iris, but it also helps in selecting the appropriate preventive healthcare measures and remedial treatments.

THE MERIDIANS

Traditional Chinese medicine, unlike Western medicine, does not rest solely on anatomical and physiological make-up. Instead, it centres around various flows of energy that travel throughout the body along specific paths (known as meridians) and in specific directions.

Until recently these energy flows were dismissed as nonsense by the orthodox medical establishment in the

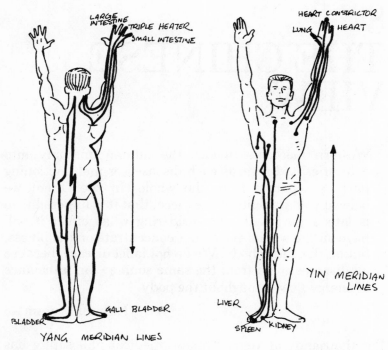

THE MERIDIANS — ENERGY CHANNELS IN THE BODY

West, despite the overwhelming historical and empirical evidence in support of the Chinese theories. For example, surgical operations have been performed for thousands of years in China with no anaesthesia other than needles piercing various points in the skin. Chinese doctors also successfully treat a seemingly endless list of medical ailments, including kidney infection, migraine, neuralgia, arthritis, constipation and skin complaints, in a like manner. However the existence of these meridians and the related forms of treatments of acupuncture and acupressure were largely ignored, along with other forms of 'alternative medicines', until their workings could be understood and proved in a laboratory. At last, a report published in 1986 by the British Medical Association accepted that the acupuncture techniques do stimulate the brain to release endorphins and encephalins, both chemicals known to help in the treatment of injuries.

The meridians can be easily tested by an electro-acupuncture machine, which will also pick out the acupuncture points along the meridians as the points of lowest electrical resistance. Furthermore, if the machine puts out a small electrical charge, it can cause a burning sensation if placed on an acupuncture point; if the machine is putting out the same electrical current but touching a different area on the skin, the burning sensation disappears immediately.

YIN AND YANG

The other basic tenet of Chinese medicine is the principle of yin and yang, which in essence means balance. Yin represents female qualities, passive, negative and cold; and yang represents the male, active, positive and hot; two subtle energies, as different as night from day and darkness from light, which together produce harmony. The whole of nature, the whole of life, depends upon the balance between these and other qualities. When the balance between these two forces is disturbed, disharmony and disorder results.

The healthy iris reflects balance, and, more particularly, balance between the body's energy flows circulating between the major organs in the body.

THE SHENG CYCLE

There are two circular flows of energy, the yin flow and the yang flow, each travelling to and from the major organs in the body, and these are particularly helpful in assessing health through the iris.

These energy flows are known as the sheng cycle, or the mother–son relationship, and they illustrate how each organ communicates with another. For instance, the cycle reveals how a problem experienced by the heart may in fact be caused by an under-functioning liver; by the same token, a continuous bladder trouble may not be the result of inherently weak bladder tissue but of lack of energy received by the bladder from the large intestines. Looked at in this way, it is easy to understand that it would be inappropriate to treat the heart or the bladder whilst the causes for the condition lay elsewhere.

The Emotional Side of the Sheng Cycle
It is certainly nothing new to suggest that different organs and areas of the body are affected by specific emotional pressures. Grief and depression, for instance, produce shallow breathing and constrict the chest and lungs, whereas anger and frustration inflame the liver. Similarly, embarrassment makes the skin become red and flushed.

But this is by no means a one-way relationship, for the condition of the different organs may produce the various emotions. Tightness of the chest may actually produce a feeling of grief and depression; in fact, one way of overcoming depression is simple by standing or sitting upright, holding the head high, opening up the chest, holding the shoulders back and by breathing deeply. And if you add a smile to this, it becomes virtually impossible to feel depressed. If you don't believe it, try it and see.

Western psychologists and researchers are slowly noticing how the body's organs are not only affected by emotions, but that they can actually create emotions. The Chinese, in contrast, have been aware of this relationship between the mind and the body for literally thousands of years, and much can be learned from their theories.

The sheng cycle therefore offers an interesting picture of a person's psychological state by looking at the interaction and functioning of the body's organs. We can see, for example, how the liver may begin to under-function when anger and frustration are experienced. Conversely, if the liver is put under physical strain, having to deal with high-fat foods, sugars, chemicals and other toxins, the person will become more prone to anger and frustration over trivial things as a result. In fact, in my own experience, it is better to avoid confrontations and arguments with

THE SHENG CYCLE

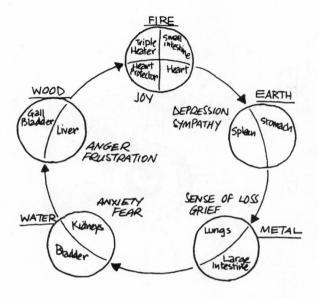

people whose eyes show disturbance in the liver, as they become loud and aggressive very quickly.

The kidneys relate to anxiety, worries and concern; because these are perhaps the most common of negative emotional states, the Chinese call the kidneys the seat of the emotions. It is not uncommon to find that a distortion of tissue in the kidney area of the right iris (between 5.30 and 6.00) is accompanied by a related disturbance diagonally opposite in the anxiety and concern zone of the head region. Therefore, when a marking appears in the anxiety and concern area in the iris, herbal remedies to flush out and cleanse the kidneys will help relieve the feelings of anxiety. A herbal infusion of buchu, elderflower, meadowsweet and comfrey is pleasant to take, either alone or with a little lemon and honey, and is an excellent formula for helping to cleanse the blood of acidity and stimulate the kidneys.

EMOTIONS AND THE SHENG CYCLE IN THE IRIS.

The spleen affects, and is affected by, chronic depression. Whenever the spleen area at 4.00 in the left iris is darkened, the person is invariably suffering from severe and chronic depression. One woman with dark brown irises visited me with her husband. Whilst she appeared to be quite jovial and outwardly relaxed, her irises told a different story. The spleen area was covered by a large dark discolouration and she had several deep tension rings with a tight nerve wreath. I asked her if there was anything in her life that was depressing her, and she then broke down in tears. It soon became apparent that she had long-standing marital and career problems which had led her to a retro-active depression. She couldn't sleep or think straight and she had been on anti-depressants and sleeping tablets for many years.

Treatment of the spleen, by either acupressure or acupuncture, or even reflexology when coupled with herbal calmatives and relaxants, often brings outstanding results in helping to overcome depression. One particular man who had the same dark colouration as the previous woman, and who had been categorised by his doctor as depressed for over 20 years, made miraculous progress. Within a period of eight weeks he was able to sleep without any tranquillisers – something he had been unable to do for years – and several months later he was able to come off the anti-depressants successfully.

When I first stumbled across it, I was absolutely amazed to notice how the iris chart correlates to the Chinese findings, but I have since found these correlations to be more and more frequent in the field of natural medicine. As far as the sheng cycle is concerned, there is little doubt in my mind that it helps us to have a more holistic view of the iris, by giving a better understanding of the possible cause and effects of dis-ease and therefore the most appropriate and effective remedies.

9
YOUR CONSTITUTION AT A GLANCE

> The most valuable aspect of Iriscopy lies in the ability to make a rapid estimation of the human constitutional disposition.
>
> Theodor Kriege, *Fundamental Basis of Irisdiagnosis*

Your constitution reflects your genetic make-up. It is the sum of your inborn physical and emotional characteristics – the general condition and character of your body. One glance at your eye reveals what type of constitution you have, whether it be a constitution showing a tendency towards a nervous disposition, one more susceptible to rheumatic and arthritic conditions, or one that is typically prone to allergies.

Most European naturopathic health practitioners who use iris analysis therefore concentrate primarily on their patients' constitutions, simply because the general constitution highlights:

- Genetic predispositions and hereditary tendencies.
- Typical symptoms affecting people with a particular constitution.
- The general preventive and remedial measures required to build on the constitutional strengths and strengthen the weaknesses.

GENETIC DISPOSITIONS AND HEREDITARY TENDENCIES

The genetic dispositions and hereditary tendencies are those tendencies and weaknesses with which we are born and which determine the type of conditions to which we are more prone. Some people have weaker or more sensitive digestive systems than others; some people are born with strong lung tissue, others are not so strong; some people are born with weak kidneys, and others have weak livers.

We all have inherent strengths and weaknesses which we carry through life, although this is not to say that we will necessarily suffer from the ailments consequent upon them. The genetic dispositions point to tendencies that we all have to certain disorders and diseases, ranging from asthma to heart disease, hay fever to skin complaints; tendencies that are passed down from parent to child. But these dispositions do not guarantee that we will suffer from these problems; they merely indicate an increased likelihood of suffering from them.

TYPICAL SYMPTOMS

An overview of the iris constitution also reflects the types of symptoms that are typically experienced over a period of time by the person, if certain lifestyle habits or environmental conditions are maintained. For instance, emotional stress affects each and every one of us, but in different ways; in one person it will lead to stomach ulcers, it will bring about a migraine in another, and a skin complaint in yet another.

The constitution therefore points to the symptoms an individual is more likely to suffer under various dietary, physical and emotional stresses. A person born with a weak stomach and a tendency to hyper-acidity is more likely to suffer stomach ulcers from nervous strain, whereas a person with poorer elimination via the skin is more likely to suffer skin complaints. The nature of the symptom will depend upon the weaker and congested body systems and organs, which all have to be taken into account when assessing a person's constitution.

Through knowledge of an individual's constitution we can thus discover not only those types of symptoms to which he or she may be more susceptible, but also the causes for those symptoms.

GENERAL PREVENTIVE AND REMEDIAL MEASURES

The general preventive and remedial healthcare measures recommended to maintain a high level of health and to avoid disease are those natural treatments and remedies

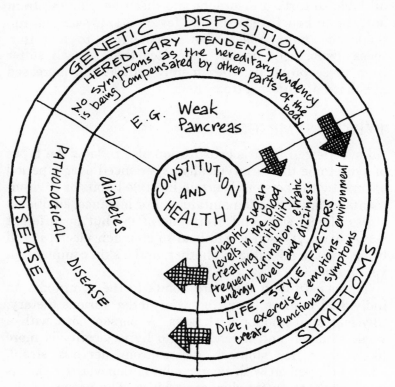

Your constitution and how it affects your health

that are designed to deal with the constitutional weaknesses. For instance, if a person has a constitution indicating that he/she is prone to hyper-acidity and related conditions (stomach ulcers, rheumatism, arthritis and minor skin complaints), he/she would be best advised to avoid altogether, or at least keep to an absolute minimum, the high acid-forming foods (e.g. meats, malt and wine vinegars, citrus fruits, wheat products, coffee, tea, alcohol, etc.). This is because acid-forming foods will only irritate the underlying tendency to accumulate acids in the body.

The accompanying flowchart shows how a knowledge of the constitution can help in a general health analysis; it shows the process of dis-ease related to our constitution. Notice how we are all born with certain genetic tendencies and specific hereditary weaknesses, although this does not mean that we will all suffer symptoms of one kind or another.

The human body is an incredible creation, very strong and quite resilient. Symptoms only follow if, after a period of time, we cause them through our lifestyle – our diet, psychological stress, lack of proper exercise, environmental toxins, climate, etc. If we choose to pursue a manner of lifestyle that puts stresses on our weaknesses, symptoms will sooner or later manifest themselves; if we do not take remedial measures to deal with the root causes of the conditions, clinical 'disease' then sets in.

THE TEN IRIS CONSTITUTIONS

The main iris types were first categorised by early German iridologists, the different categories of constitutions being determined by the different colours and structures and therefore reflecting the functional and structural constitutional strengths and weaknesses.

Whilst every one of us is unique, most people fall into one or more of the various categories of constitutions. It is therefore not uncommon to find that a person's irises cannot be categorised solely into one constitutional type but are instead a combination of two or more constitutional types. However, if we concentrate on the main

THE CONSTITUTIONS

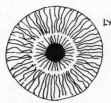
LYMPHATIC

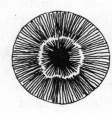
LYMPHATIC NEUROGENIC

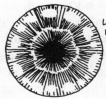
LYMPHATIC HYDROGENOID

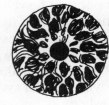
LYMPHATIC CONNECTIVE TISSUE WEAKNESS

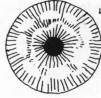
LYMPHATIC URIC ACID DIATHESIS

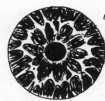
LYMPHATIC ABDOMINAL RESERVOIR

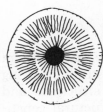
LIPAEMIC DIATHESIS

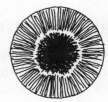
BILIARY

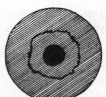
HAEMATOGENIC

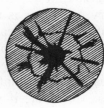
HAEMATOGENIC ANXIETY TETANIC

features of an iris, these categories do give us an excellent overall health analysis at a quick glance, and they also indicate general preventive measures that should be considered in order to maintain health and avoid disease.

LYMPHATIC CONSTITUTION

The pure lymphatic constitution type is a blue/grey iris with loose wavy fibres. The genetic tendencies are hyper-acidity (particularly in the alimentary tract), and an irritable lymphatic system. Typical conditions suffered by people with this constitution include acidity in the stomach and intestines, arthritis, rheumatism, skin complaints, allergies, swollen glands and ulcers.

Remedial Measures
If you fall within this category the following measures would be recommended.

Diet Avoid high acid-forming foods, and be sure to balance acid/alkaline foods carefully in the diet (see anti-acid diet on page 264) so that the acid levels in the blood and tissues do not reach high levels.

Exercise Take regular exercise to help stimulate the flow of lymph and avoid lymphatic congestion.

Footbaths Take hot and cold footbaths to encourage blood and lymph circulation (see page 90).

Skin brushing Daily skin brushing removes dead skin cells and improves elimination of toxins through the skin. This also helps blood and lymph circulation (see page 90).

Relax Don't allow anxiety, worries or resentment to build up; even if we eat the best foods in the world, the body will create acidity through these emotions.

The functioning of the kidneys in filtering acids from

the bloodstream is particularly affected by these emotions. Chinese medical philosophy has maintained for thousands of years that the kidneys are the seat of the emotions. You may have noticed how, in the iris chart, the anxiety and concern area is diagonally opposite the kidney and adrenal glands.

LYMPHATIC-NEUROGENIC CONSTITUTION

The lymphatic-neurogenic type is a blue/grey base colour and characterised by elongated fine fibres of silk-linen structure. Whilst physiologically strong, this type of person has excess nervous energy and is apt to put the central and autonomic nervous system under strain by worrying about trivial matters and getting uptight and worked up too easily. A lymphatic-neurogenic person does not find it easy to relax, and often keeps him/herself busy due to the excess nervous energy. The person has a high pain threshold and often continues without listening to his/her body until eventually a health crisis occurs.

Typical disorders to which a person with a lymphatic-neurogenic constitution would be more prone include headache / migraines, ulcers, nervous disorders, arthritis and rheumatism, and skin complaints.

Remedial Measures
If you fall within this category the following preventive measures are recommended.

Avoid stimulants Avoid nerve stimulants such as tea, coffee, alcohol, and foods or soft drinks containing refined sugars, all of which will deplete the body of vitamin B complex – which is food for the nervous system – and will therefore make the nervous system less able to cope with high levels of stress.

Avoid heavy workloads Avoid prolonged heavy workloads without taking time in the day to relax. A lymphatic-neurogenic person tends to be on the go continually throughout the day, and this allows tensions to accumulate in the body. It would be far more beneficial to find a form of relaxation that you enjoy, in order to give the nervous system a rest and to calm down the body systems. Do this on a regular basis.

Avoid refined foods Avoid refined foods (e.g. white bread, cakes, sugar, etc.). In order to metabolise these foods (i.e. to convert them into energy) the body needs the nutrients that are normally found in the whole food in nature, most of which are removed from the food in the refining process. Therefore when we eat refined foods the body has to use up those vital nutrients from its own tissues in order to convert the food into energy. Rather than nourishing the body we are instead slowly but surely, depleting it of its reserves. Refined foods therefore only serve further to weaken the nervous system, and indeed the entire body.

Avoid acid foods Avoid high acid-forming foods and ensure acid/alkaline foods are carefully balanced in the diet (see anti-acid diet on page 264) so that the acid levels in the blood and tissues do not reach high levels.

Keep active Keep physically active and mobile to ensure flexibility of the joints. The connective tissue is already tight, and lack of exercise can lead to the joints seizing up. Whilst people in this category always tend instinctively to be on the go, rushing about from here to there, this is not a complete form of exercise. It is therefore important to exercise and stretch the joints and the whole of the body in order to maintain a healthy physical balance.

Keep within your limits Keep a mental check on your lifestyle. Have you heard of people who never take a day off sick from work in their lives and then die suddenly from a heart attack or cancer? It is more often than not lymphatic-neurogenic type of persons that this happens to; being of a strong physiological constitution, they have a tendency to go beyond their physical limits without realising it, until a crisis occurs. They tend to ignore minor ailments and symptoms without taking time to listen to the needs of their bodies.

LYMPHATIC-HYDROGENOID CONSTITUTION

The lymphatic-hydrogenoid type is again a blue/grey base colour iris, categorised by white-orange puffy clouds around the periphery of the iris. This indicates congestion of the lymphatic vessels and fluid retention. The darker the colour of the 'puffs', the more chronic the congestion in the lymph vessels.

Typical disorders affecting people with this type of constitution include swollen glands, hayfever, allergies, sinusitis, oedema (water retention) and persistent infections.

Remedial Measures

Avoid mucus-forming foods It is important to avoid mucus-forming foods (e.g. meats, chocolates, dairy foods such as milk, cheeses, etc., sugars, fatty foods), as these put additional strain on the already overburdened and congested lymphatic system. Dairy foods are particularly harmful and are best avoided as far as possible.

Instead eat plenty of raw fruits and salads (although not at the same meal, as the acids do not combine well), and lightly steamed root and green vegetables. The bulk of the diet (50–70 per cent) should consist of these foods as they are nourishing and have a cleansing effect on the blood and lymph systems.

Encourage blood/lymph circulation Encourage blood and lymph circulation through:

- Regular daily exercise. A brisk 20-minute walk or swim, jogging or cycling in the park, or 15 minutes on a bouncer (a small exercise trampoline) are all excellent forms of exercise, involving muscular activity all over the body. Whatever the form of exercise, ensure that it is something that will make the heart beat a little faster and produce perspiration. This way it will ensure that the heart muscle is kept strong, the lymph is kept flowing by the contraction of the muscle tissues, and elimination of body wastes through the skin in perspiration is encouraged.

- Hot and cold footbaths (see page 87). This is one of the oldest forms of hydrotherapy, for, apart from improving blood and lymph flow, they tone and strengthen the body. Hot and cold footbaths help break up crystals that develop on the nerve endings in the feet which are considered by reflexologists to affect other parts of the body. Those crystal deposits are then taken back into the bloodstream and eliminated. In fact this home treatment has been so effective over the centuries that many naturopaths as well as reflexologists advise all their patients to take alternate hot and cold footbaths to supplement and assist the naturopathic and reflexology treatments.
- Daily skin brushing (see pages 263–4). Again this improves circulation, and also helps eliminate dead skin cells.
- Saunas are also an excellent way of helping the body eliminate toxins through the skin and improving circulation.
- Body massage. Remedial massage is the oldest form of physical therapy and one of the most effective ways, not only to calm and soothe the nervous system, but also to stimulate blood and lymph circulation and cleanse the body tissues. Tests I have conducted in my clinic have shown conclusively that the ketones (waste chemicals) in the urine are a lot higher after having had a massage than at any other time. This means that more waste is being eliminated from the body.

Deep breathing　It is known that deep breathing exercises encourage elimination of toxins through the lungs and prevent the build-up of mucus in the respiratory tract.

However deep breathing also relaxes the body and is one of the most effective ways of stimulating the lymphatic system. (One of the reasons why people turn to cigarettes in times of stress is that the process of smoking forces them to take deep breaths, even though the air they inhale is polluted with known carcinogens such as nicotine and benzopyrene.)

Dr Jack Shields, a lymphologist from Santa Barbara, California, concluded from his studies that deep diaphragmatic breathing when coupled with physical exercise can accelerate the cleansing of the lymphatic system by as much as 15 times.

Avoid acid foods Again, avoid high acid-forming foods and ensure that acid/alkaline foods are carefully balanced in the diet in order to avoid the build up of acidity in the body (see page 264).

LYMPHATIC ABDOMINAL RESERVOIR CONSTITUTION

The lymphatic abdominal reservoir constitution type is a blue/grey iris characterised by an enlarged and ballooned A.N.W. and usually accompanied by several lacunae. It shows a weakened digestive and hormonal system and a sluggish intestinal tract.

The main weakness in this constitution is the lack of tone in the wall of the large intestine and a weakened autonomic nervous system. Typical symptoms include gastrointestinal disturbances (colitis, irritable bowels, haemorrhoids), nervous disorders and hormonal imbalance.

Remedial Measures

Eat a high fibre wholefood diet This will encourage regular bowel movements; if necessary, take one level teaspoon of psyllium husk with a large glass of water before each meal to add soft soluble bulk to the diet.

Avoid processed and refined foods These foods serve to weaken the tissue further. For instance, to metabolise white sugar one needs the vital nutrients, minerals and vitamins which would come with it in its natural state. As these vital nutrients are missing from the refined food, the body will take those elements from its own tissue and therefore deplete its vital reserves.

Exercise regularly Do regular daily exercise paying particular attention to the abdominal muscles to help restore tone to the tissues surrounding the colon.

LIPAEMIC DIATHESIS CONSTITUTION

The lipaemic diathesis constitution is characterised by a sodium/cholesterol ring going around the outer edge of the iris indicating a tendency to hardening of the arteries and a build up of cholesterol and/or mineral deposits.

The main health problems associated with this type of constitution are of course the excess cholesterol and minerals (calcium and sodium) in the body that lead to hardening of the arteries and arthritis due to the excess calcium deposits in and around the joints.

Remedial Measures

Avoid high fat foods All meats, poultry, chocolates, fried foods, dairy foods (especially full fat and hard cheeses), i.e. those foods which contain high amounts of fat and cholesterol.

Eat foods that help cleanse the bloodstream Plenty of water-rich foods (fresh fruits, vegetables, sprouted seeds), pulses, onions, garlic and lecithin supplements all help rid the body of excess fats and cholesterol.

Exercise regularly Take up daily exercise to keep the joints mobile and flexible and encourage good blood circulation.

Avoid all mineral supplements These are often poorly assimilated by the body and may form deposits in and around the joints.

Take cleansing drinks Drink plenty (one or two glasses daily) of distilled water and/or raw fresh fruit and vegetable juices which also help cleanse the body of toxins and dissolve accumulations inside the body.

LYMPHATIC-URIC ACID DIATHESIS CONSTITUTION

The lymphatic-uric acid diathesis type has a blue/grey iris characterised by a thickened nerve wreath near to the pupil, and white puffy clouds around the central areas of the iris rather than the outer edges as in the lymphatic-hydrogenoid constitution mentioned above. It indicates retention of uric acid in the tissues and weak kidney function.

Typical disorders to which people with this type of constitution are more prone include gout, rheumatism, arthritis, fibrositis and kidney stones.

Remedial Measures

Avoid protein- and acid-rich foods Avoid high protein- and high acid-forming foods (see page 264), especially meats and poultry, dairy foods, salt, processed flour products, coffee, tea and alcohol, as the urea and uric acid produced by these foods put strain on the kidneys. Furthermore when muscles exercise they produce lactic acid as a waste product, and this forms crystals when combined with uric acid. Therefore high levels of uric acid in the diet can lead to high levels of acid crystals in the tissues, and it is these acid crystals that cause pain in rheumatic and arthritic disorders.

Instead, eat plenty of fresh fruits (except citrus fruits), salads, and vegetables, and drink their freshly squeezed juices, all of which have a cleansing and alkalising effect on the blood and tissues.

Exercise regularly Do regular exercise to keep the joints and surrounding tissues flexible and to avoid stiffness. Light aerobic exercises are better than heavy body-building exercises as the faster lighter exercises encourage deeper breathing and produce the consequent elimination of carbonic acid through the lungs.

Cut down on alcohol Avoid putting excessive strain on the kidneys through alcohol consumption; limit yourself to four units each week (half a pint of beer or 1 oz. liquor is a unit). The kidneys filter acids from the blood stream and the more strain they are put under, the less efficient they will be in cleansing the blood. Drinking a lot of water is not a remedy for excessive alcohol consumption and will probably only augment the problem because more fluid in the body means more work for the kidneys in filtering it.

Body massage Remedial massage is the oldest form of physical therapy and one of the most effective ways, not only to calm and soothe the nervous system, but also to stimulate blood and lymph circulation and cleanse the body tissues.

LYMPHATIC-CONNECTIVE TISSUE WEAKNESS CONSTITUTION

The lymphatic-connective tissue weakness type again has a blue/grey base coloured iris with loosely connected iris fibres resembling a spider's web and having a hessian-net structure.

This constitution type is physiologically weak, with weak connective tissue throughout the body. A person with this constitution therefore generally takes longer to recuperate than other types. Whilst again being more prone to acid conditions, this type has a genetic predisposition to spinal and joint weakness of the ligaments and tendons, varicose veins, haemorrhoids, prolapse, joint displacement and general under-functioning of the visceral organs.

Remedial Measures

Avoid processed/refined foods Avoid processed and refined foods, which will only weaken the tissue further. To metabolise white sugar, for instance, one needs the vital nutrients, minerals and vitamins that would normally be present in its natural state. As these vital nutrients are missing from the refined food, the body will take elements from its own tissue in order to metabolise the food, and will therefore deplete its own vital reserves.

Exercise regularly Do regular daily exercise, particularly isometric exercises – the most effective exercise to strengthen tissue (see page 237) – and ensure that the posture is correct so that blood and nerve supply are unrestricted.

Tissue strength depends upon a good blood supply, to transport the nutrients to the tissue and take away the cell wastes, and an unhindered nerve supply, to create muscular contraction. If either blood or nerve supply is faulty the part of the body affected will degenerate.

Ensure adequate nutrition Strength of tissue is dependent upon receiving vital nutrients, and these must therefore be present in the diet. Wholefoods, raw fruits and vegetables, and sprouted seeds and legumes are all cleansing and highly nutritious, being packed with vitamins, minerals and enzymes that can be easily assimilated by the body.

Keep the bowels regular Ensure the bowels are moving daily by having plenty of fibre in the diet, taking regular exercise, and trying to let go of past hurts/memories; holding on to unresolved emotional conflicts causes the bowels to tighten and hold the waste matter inside.

BILIARY CONSTITUTION

The biliary iris is brown/hazel, overlaid (usually around the pupil) on a blue/green base. This type of constitution has a genetic predisposition to gastro-intestinal weakness, with poor liver/gall bladder and pancreas function, and an easily strained autonomic nervous system.

Typical conditions affecting people with this type of constitution include biliousness, digestive disorders, including flatulance and constipation, lethargy, erratic blood sugar levels, migraines and skin complaints.

Remedial Measures

Avoid fatty and sugary foods Avoid high fat foods, fried foods and meats. High sugar foods should also be avoided as they will ferment in the alimentary tract, adding to the already high levels of toxicity.

Ensure adequate nutrition Ensure the diet is rich with raw fruits and vegetables, and wholegrains (e.g. brown rice, oats, barley, millet and buckwheat), as these foods are cleansing, nourishing and easier to digest.

Keep the bowels regular Ensure the bowels move daily, and take regular exercise to encourage a peristaltic movement of the bowels.

Furthermore, have a regular annual bowel cleanse to ensure the bowels move smoothly and to prevent the build up of toxins within the alimentary tract (see pages 167–8 and 200).

No alcohol Avoid alcohol, as this puts stress on the liver and kidneys. These are two of the major elimination organs in the body, and any excessive strain on these will ultimately lead to poor elimination of toxins from the system.

Deep breathing Deep breathing exercises (see page 149) are important to calm and soothe the nervous system and also to help cleanse the body of waste through the lymphatic system.

HAEMATOGENIC CONSTITUTION

The haematogenic type is a pure brown base coloured iris with radials from the pupil or nerve wreath. This type often has hereditary weaknesses in the blood-making mechanisms, poor endocrine (hormonal) function, digestive disorders, and poor elimination through the bowels and skin.

Typical conditions affecting people with this type of constitution include blood disorders (anemia), digestive disorders, biliousness, stomach cramps, and premenstrual tension in women.

Remedial Measure

Avoid fatty and processed foods Avoid tea, coffee and alcohol, chocolates, meats, fried foods and dairy foods (especially full-fat and hard cheeses). These foods thicken the blood and add large amounts of toxins, and therefore unnecessary strain, to the digestive system.

Avoid processed foods and those with chemical additives as these put a strain on the liver.

Eat water-rich foods Eat plenty of water-rich foods (fresh fruits, vegetables, and sprouted seeds and legumes) as these are highly nourishing, easily digested and very cleansing.

Deep breathing Stimulate elimination through the lungs and lymph via the regular use of deep breathing exercises

Keep the bowels regular Ensure the bowels move daily, and take regular exercise to encourage the peristaltic movement of the bowels.

Have a regular annual bowel cleanse to prevent the build up of toxins within the alimentary tract (see pages 167-168).

Keep the organs of elimination healthy Ensure that the other eliminating organs (lungs, lymph, kidneys and skin), particularly the skin, are functioning well. Stimulate elimination through the skin by skin brushing, saunas and regular exercise producing perspiration.

HAEMATOGENIC ANXIETY-TETANIC CONSTITUTION

This constitution is similar to the haematogenic iris type, a brown base colour iris with radials. However there are also tension rings, indicating hyper-active neuromuscular activity, and a tendency towards psychosomatic disorders, gastro-intestinal disorders, blood disorders and glandular disorders.

Typical disorders affecting people with this type of constitution include anxiety, hypertension, tension headaches, and gastro-intestinal disturbances including constipation and irritable bowels.

Remedial Measures

Avoid fatty and processed foods Avoid meats, processed foods, tea, coffee and alcohol, chocolates, fried foods, dairy foods (especially full-fat and hard cheeses); these are foods that thicken the blood and introduce large amounts of toxins, putting unnecessary strain on the digestive system.

Eat water-rich foods Eat plenty of water-rich foods (fresh fruits, vegetables, and sprouted seeds and legumes) as these are highly nourishing, easily digested and very cleansing.

Deep breathing Do deep breathing exercises to calm and soothe the nervous system and stimulate elimination through the lungs and lymph.

Keep the bowels regular Ensure the bowels move daily and take regular exercise to encourage the peristaltic movement of the bowels.

Furthermore, have a regular annual bowel cleanse to prevent the build up of toxins within the alimentary tract (see pages 167–8).

Reduce negative emotions Sort out negative emotions, which are often the cause of the digestive and other disturbances affecting people with this type of constitution.

Take up a relaxation technique to prevent the build up of emotional strain.

10
EYE DISORDERS AND DISEASES

> The origin of eye diseases is the general bodily condition of the individual sufferer, and his past medical history.
>
> Harry Benjamin, *Better Sight Without Glasses*

No organ functions in isolation but is always dependent upon the functioning of other parts of the body, and nowhere in the human body is this more true than in the case of the eye.

The eye is one of the most sensitive and delicate organs of the human body. It requires more oxygen than any other organ in the body. Furthermore, its health can only be assured when there is an unrestricted flow of blood and unhindered nerve supply; where either of these is absent the function and substance of the eye will suffer.

In using the iris as a means of health assessment, eye diseases and disorders are particularly important, not only because many are actually caused by general bodily functions, but because the disorders and diseases themselves often affect the iris and eye tissues. When the iris is affected, other parts of the body will, in turn, suffer.

MYOPIA AND HYPERMETROPIA

For instance, shortsightedness (myopia) is a common complaint in which the eyeball and/or lens becomes distorted in shape due to the imbalance of the muscles around it. It is mostly an acquired condition caused from continuous close-up work or reading, which puts certain eye muscles into spasm for long periods of time; the muscles find it difficult to relax, and consequently the eye cannot adjust to focus on images in the distance. A student may read for hours at a time and then look up to see something in the distance but find everything further than say, 10 yards away is blurred and out of focus.

Hypermetropia (farsightedness) is likewise often associated with imbalanced muscle tissues around the eyeball. Both hypermetropia and myopia often result in strain on the eye muscles, and lead to headaches and migraine. But at the same time the eye will often squint and the iris fibres will contract, reducing the size of the pupil in order to produce a sharper image for the retina. This process will produce tension in the tissues in and around the eye, and indeed throughout the body, and may result in further symptoms including giddiness, nausea, and vomiting. Therefore to eliminate the headaches and any other symptoms, the person will need more than painkillers or even tranquillisers and relaxants; to get at the root of the problem, something must be done about the eye strain.

It is for this reason that the renowned Bate's method of correcting eyesight disturbances by relaxing, re-balancing and re-educating the eye tissues often corrects not only defective vision but other disorders, ranging from migraine to fibrositis and indigestion – problems which at first sight might appear to be totally unconnected to the original eye strain.

CATARACT

Cataract is a disease affecting the lens in the eye, which becomes clogged with residue and waste products of inefficient metabolism. In the process, the crystalline lens becomes opaque and prevents light from entering the eyeball. If left untreated, cataract leads to blindness. Many people suffering from diabetes go on to develop a cataract, as do a large number of people who suffer from Bright's disease. This underlines the suggestion that the cause of the cataract is closely connected with the overall health of the bloodstream.

As the lens lies behind the iris, a cataract leaves the iris fibres very much unaffected and therefore has little relevance to an iris analysis. The iris remains clearly visible and undisturbed. However during the course of an iris analysis, if the pupil appears grey in colour it is advisable to consult an ophthalmologist immediately for a diagnosis, and to commence a general cleansing health programme, as the cataract is only a reflection of much more deep-seated health problems. Indeed, in the bestselling book *Better Sight Without Glasses* Harry Benjamin cites several patient case histories as examples of how a cataract discovered in its early stages can, through a cleansing diet and natural treatments, entirely disappear, and even chronic cataract may be prevented from worsening.

GLAUCOMA

Glaucoma is a disorder of the eye in which pressure builds up within the eyeball due to the accumulation of excess fluid. The eyeball becomes hard, the faulty drainage and congestion of fluid in the eye pushes the iris forward and the lens appears opaque, with a green tinge to it. The condition is usually treated surgically by making an incision into the iris itself, to allow fluid to escape from the eyeball and so relieve the pressure. However, whilst this helps the patient's eyesight (at least in the short term), the removal of a section of the iris may have serious implications for the patient's general well-being.

Removal of a section of an iris will affect the tissues in the related part of the body. Generally, glaucoma operations are carried out to the upper half of an iris, so that in day-to-day affairs it is not easily noticeable and therefore will not cause embarrassment to the patient. However, as you will recall, the upper half of the iris mainly relates to the head, and several cases have been reported of people having disturbed sleep patterns, or suffering increased anxiety, reduced memory and even of becoming epileptic, after a glaucoma operation. The nature of the problem will of course depend upon the precise section of the iris that has been removed.

I remember examining one man's irises and discovering that a wedge had been removed from the right iris between approximately 10.00 and 10.10 (a triangular wedge pointing inwards from the sclera is the typical sign of a glaucoma operation). I asked him if he had had any trouble with the right side of his neck and shoulder, and he then proceeded to tell me that this was his main problem and had been for the past six years. He had a continuous ache and a numbness around the region, which had not been helped by physiotherapy or painkilling drugs, and all the standard hospital tests could find nothing wrong with the joints or the muscle tissues.

So I asked him how long ago he had had the glaucoma operation, and he said about six years or so. I then asked him if he could remember which came first, the glaucoma operation or the shoulder problem, and he replied without hesitation that the operation had been carried out four months before the onset of his shoulder pains. It was only then that he first considered the possibility that the persistent ache in his neck might have been connected with his glaucoma operation. However, now that the section of iris had been removed very little could be done except regular reflexology treatments which work through the nervous system and help counter the damaged nerve reflexes in the iris.

Like most eye diseases and disorders, glaucoma is a symptom of a greater underlying cause. One British psychologist, J.M. Heaton, in his book *The Eye*, linked chronic depressions with glaucoma. Naturopaths have contended for years that glaucoma is constitutional in character and therefore requires constitutional treatment of the entire body and particularly the elimination systems as the first course of action (except in severe cases), in preference to local surgery.

11
REFLECTIONS OF EYES

The patients are your textbooks.
The sick bed is your study.

Paracelcus

Every time I look into someone's eyes I learn something
new and often something very precious, for every eye is
different and tells a different story. I have been very
fortunate indeed to have become aware of this ancient
science of iris analysis, for my patients have been my
teachers. They have taught me not just about the different
ways the eyes reflect the conditions of the body, and not
just about the practice of natural health care: they have
taught me much about myself and about life.

The following cases serve to illustrate the value of iris
analysis in assessing a person's physical and emotional
health and the process of change it can produce in life.

MRS L

I saw Mrs L on only one occasion, and have never seen her
since. She had been referred to me by her son for a specific
problem that had badly affected the sight in her right eye.

Mrs L had only recently recovered from Bell's palsy
(facial paralysis) that had affected the movement of the
muscles in the right side of her face. Whilst she was now
free of most of the related symptoms, and was, for
instance, able to talk, smile and eat easily, there still
remained one important difficulty – to open her right eye.
The palsy had left her with a dropped right eyelid, and try
what she may, she could not open it.

She had had all the standard medical tests, none of which had thrown any light on the matter. Her doctor and the specialists she had consulted had all told her the same story; the nerve was practically dead, was unlikely to recover, and there was therefore nothing that could be done. She should be grateful that she was still able to use one eye – she could quite easily get by with it if she tried.

A quick glance at her eyes revealed a cholesterol ring, indicating hardening of the arteries, particularly marked in the head and facial zones, and a spastic colon with toxic congestion affecting the nerve wreath, which, although jagged in places, was not broken. The nerve was therefore unlikely to be dead, so there was hope.

I then asked Mrs L to blink her eyes as fast as she could. Her left eyelid moved rapidly, while the right eyelid was flickering slightly despite the fact that Mrs L had been told that the nerve on the right side of her face was as good as dead. It was therefore fair to assume the nerve was not totally dead. However, as the problem had obviously taken a long time to develop, it would therefore probably take some time to go. During the consultation Mrs L mentioned that she had had poor bowel movements and that she was of a nervous disposition. She also recalled noticing, and being told by her optician as far back as eight years previously, that her right eyelid was very slightly drooping.

I immediately advised her to go on a low-cholesterol high-fibre diet, with plenty of fresh fruit and vegetable juices, and lecithin supplements to break down cholesterol deposits in the arteries. On top of that, I recommended that she palm her eyes (a method of gently massaging the eyes) to relax the surrounding tissues and improve blood circulation in the area. I also advised a course of reflexology treatment, but as Mrs L had been unable to find a reflexologist in her locality I showed her husband how to treat the nerve reflexes in his wife's feet to stimulate the nerves in and around the eye.

Three weeks later I was informed through a mutual friend that Mrs L's eyelid had begun to move almost half

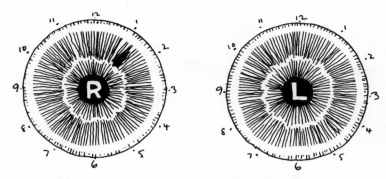

*Mrs L – conquering the effects of Bell's palsy
(facial paralysis)*

of the way back towards its normal position. Another two months passed before I received a call from Mrs L herself to let me know that her eyelid had fully opened in its correct position and was functioning properly.

MR C

Mr C visited me after reading an article about my practice and my development of the video-iriscope. He had an extremely likeable manner, and after explaining the basic principles of iris analysis I filmed his eyes in the usual way and proceeded with a verbal analysis.

It was obvious that he had a lymphatic-uric acid diathesis constitution, so his main troubles were likely to lie with hyper-acidity, particularly in the muscular/ skeletal system. The eyes do not record symptoms, but he had such a prevalence of white clouds (inflammation) in the muscular/skeletal zones that I suspected he was getting rheumatic pain, and it later transpired that he was indeed suffering acute pain.

As we have mentioned, every condition will have two causes, an underlying cause and an explosive cause. In the case of Mr C, he had an acid constitution and a build up of acidity, added to which the autonomic nerve wreath was broken at 1.30 in the left iris, indicating a nerve restriction

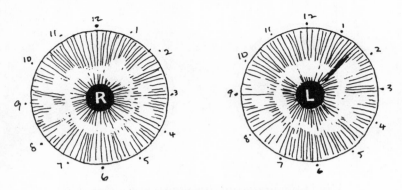

Mr C – chronic pains in the neck

in the middle of the neck (cervical vertebrae 3–5).

Mr C then admitted that he was in intense pain most of the time and particularly in his neck and upper back. Ten years previously he had been attacked and badly beaten, and kicked in the upper back and neck. It was since then that he had been suffering intense pain. Visits to hospitals and specialists showed nothing, until two weeks prior to seeing me tests had finally confirmed damage to the nerve root between cervical vertebrae 3 and 4.

The general acidity could be helped by an anti-acid diet and herbal remedies, but Mr C really needed structural treatment for his neck. However, until the acidity was reduced the area was too tender even to touch.

MRS M

Mrs M attended a lecture I had given in London, and then made an appointment to see me. The dark brown eyes with tension rings and deep radials showed a haematogenic anxiety-tetanic constitution, and it was clear she had accumulated a lot of stress, while the narrow autonomic nerve wreath indicated a tightness in the intestines. However the rest of the irides were clear except for a small discolouration between 3.00 and 4.00 in the left iris, indicating lymphatic congestion in the left breast.

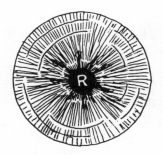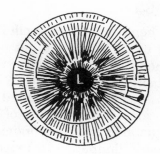

Mrs M – cancer of the left breast

It transpired that she had suffered from chronic constipation caused from long-standing emotional stress – she resented her husband. However, the main reason why she had decided to come to see me was that six months previously she had had a malignant growth removed from her left breast. Since the operation she had been having homoeopathic treatment to rebuild the body's defences, and she now wanted to see if the left breast area was clear.

All I could do in such a case was to reassure her that the remaining condition in the tissue would eventually go if she continued a cleansing programme. Whilst Mrs M was taking homoeopathic treatments, I stressed that all tablets, whether herbal, homoeopathic or allopathic, were not 'cures'; they could be crutches, helping the body in times of crisis, but health cannot be created without healthy living – dietary, structural, emotional and spiritual. Furthermore, although diet is crucial to health, cleansing the body does not just involve dietary changes. It also involves cleansing the emotions and looking at the physical structure.

Mrs M would therefore have to resolve her inner emotional conflicts and let go of her anger and bitterness, especially relating to her husband. Then the real cleansing process could begin.

MRS H

When I first set up a clinic with a leading optometrist Mrs H came to see me out of curiosity. She was a personal friend of my colleague and was interested to know more about iris analysis.

Mrs H's irises showed a lymphatic neurogenic constitution, with a build up of acidity throughout the body and a defined scurf rim indicating poor blood circulation and poor elimination through the skin. However, when I mentioned this to her she was not very happy about the analysis as she felt very fit and healthy. She kept to what she considered to be a good balanced diet and exercised daily in a gym. As far as she was aware she had no evidence of acidity and her circulation seemed fine; after all, she didn't get cold hands and feet. (People with excess acidity often don't experience cold extremities because the high acid levels cause inflammation and thus heat.) She also had had no skin complaints other than an itchy rash under her armpits several months previously, but that had been 'cured' by antibiotics.

Mrs H was therefore quite reluctant to follow a dietary regimen and a course of herbal remedies; as far as she was concerned she had no problem. A year later. however, she paid me another visit and recounted her story. Approximately four months after seeing me her skin condition had come back with a vengeance, covering most of her body and causing widespread itching. She had been to see a Chinese herbalist whose herbal preparations had helped,

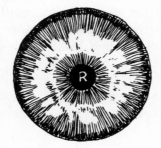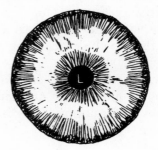

Mrs H – skin eruptions

and she had also gone on to a strict diet based on allergy testing. This had also helped, but she still had the condition. What could I suggest?

On this second visit her acid levels were much higher than the year before. She therefore needed to go on an anti-acid diet, with herbal remedies to stimulate the kidneys and naturopathic treatments to stimulate elimination of acids through the skin.

MS A, A YOUNG GIRL

Ms A was a small six-year-old child whose eyes showed a lymphatic constitution, with weak tissue in the legs, kidneys and neck. She had been suffering from pains in the legs, with a high temperature, and inflammation in her neck which came on every six weeks. This had continued for the past six months, despite continuous use of antibiotics.

I suggested that we remove all the major acid-forming foods from her diet, that she should take herbal remedies and tissue salts to assist the kidneys' elimination of acids, while at the same time improving her blood circulation with hot and cold footbaths. Within two months the symptoms had all but disappeared; we had simply identified the weak areas and the levels of congestion, and treated her condition accordingly.

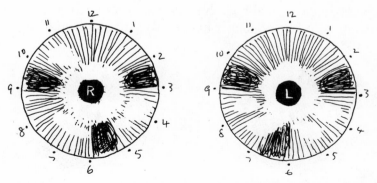

Ms A – overcoming fevers, infections and pains in the legs

The photographs show how her irides changed during the succeeding six months, with a great reduction in the acidity and the slight knitting together of the fibres in the areas relating to the neck and kidneys.

MR W

A bright white halo around the pupil and a brightness of the autonomic nerve wreath clearly showed that Mr H had severe hyper-acidity in his intestinal tract. Indeed, this was a condition that he had had for many years, and that he only kept under control with strong medications – he had been on steroids for over six years. However the symptoms were only being suppressed, and he was still bleeding from his rectum.

Mr W had deep-seated family stresses, with irritation from his wife, and his job involved him travelling around the country. Often he would have to eat whatever he could get, and whatever he could get was usually junk food and high acid-forming foods, which only served to aggravate the acid condition.

All I could do was to help him out with the physical side of his complaint. I advised him to keep as best he could to an anti-acid diet (see pages 264–5), and gave him slippery elm to soothe the internal inflammations and absorb the excess acidity. Herbal remedies to help the kidneys eliminate the build up of acids, together with raw vegetable juices of cabbage and carrot, produced wonderful results, until he no longer needed the steroid preparations.

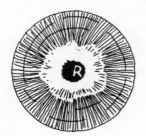 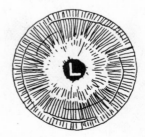

Mr W – the picture of ulcers

However the condition did not reverse totally because he still refused to confront or deal with his marital problems. It was even plain to him that the emotional factors were very important, because the condition flared up at times when he and his wife renewed old disagreements. These also affected the children of the family, all of whom had deep tension rings in their eyes.

MR P

Mr P was a Belgian living in London. I was treating him for backache when one day he visited my clinic, complaining that he was feeling well below par. He had been to his medical doctor in Belgium about this only a week earlier, but had been told to take a few aspirin. Although he was run down, he had been told there was nothing wrong with him.

One look in his eyes revealed weak and inflamed tissue in the lungs and bronchials. He was a heavy smoker, but did not want to give this up or stick to a full naturopathic programme, because he had no real incentive to do so; after all, he had no symptoms such as a chesty cough relating to this area. I remained adamant, however, and insisted that at the very least he should visit his medical doctor in London and ask for a thorough examination. Later that week I received a letter from him telling me that he had visited his doctor the day after he had seen me, and that he had been diagnosed as having bronchial pneumonia.

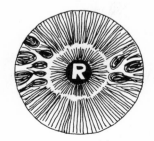 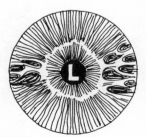

Mr P – bronchial problems

JASON, A LITTLE BOY

Central toxaemia is a common condition these days, typically poor Western diets and prolific use of antibiotics contributing to a build up of toxicity in the intestinal tract. Whilst symptoms are generally not easily seen through the eyes, in this case you can be sure that any person with central toxaemia will be suffering not only from conditions relating to the intestines, but also from general lethargy because nutrients are being inefficiently absorbed through the small intestines.

Jason was a ten-year-old boy whose eyes showed an extremely dark intestinal zone, one of the darkest cases of central toxaemia I have ever seen. I mentioned the condition to his mother, who said that he had been suffering from chronic lethargy and it had now reached the stage where he could not concentrate in lessons at school and he had no energy to play games or sports. I asked what his typical diet was, and whether he had had any prolonged use of antibiotics in his life, and amazing as it might seem, discovered he had had antibiotics for the first full year of his life. Even if he had been eating the best foods in the world he would not have absorbed the nutrients efficiently, as antibiotics kill off the internal flora found in the intestines and thereby allow a toxic environment to develop.

We immediately put Jason on a basic cleansing diet,

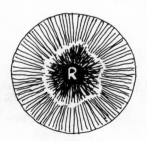 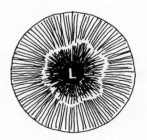

Jason – beating chronic fatigue

with a herbal detoxification formula to stimulate the liver to help flush out the accumulated toxicity, and tissue salts to help the body deal more efficiently with the nutrients it had absorbed. These were accompanied by basic hot and cold footbaths to act as a gentle tonic and to encourage blood circulation. Slowly we were able to build on this with Chinese moxibustion to stimulate the body's energy channels and the major elimination channels.

Six months later I was invited to dinner by Jason's mother. The whole family were present and Jason looked spritely and fresh. I will always remember how, during the last course of dinner, Jason, who had been sitting next to me, leant over and whispered 'Thank you for helping me not to be tired anymore'.

MR R

Mr R walked into my clinic on a Sunday morning. He had been referred to me by a local naturopath for a complete iris analysis, as this was to form the basis of the naturopath's treatment programme.

But I didn't need to look into Mr R's eyes to realise that he was seriously ill; his complexion was sallow, with a pale-grey pallor, and he moved uneasily. His iris analysis confirmed my suspicions. He had a large build up of

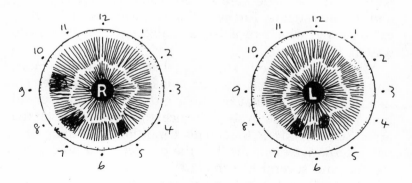

Mr R – picking up the problem undetected by x-rays

toxicity, particularly around his liver and bladder, both of which showed weak and degenerate tissue. He also had a large and extremely bright arcus senilis, indicating more than just hardening of the arteries, for the brightness of the ring indicated inflammation in the blood and lymph systems. When I examined the left iris an even more serious condition became apparent; the dark black discolouration at 6.15 in the intestinal zone indicated a blockage and deep congestion in the tissues of the upper rectum.

After the analysis he informed me that he had had cancer of the liver, for which he was presently being treated. He had also had cancer of the bladder five years earlier, the bladder having been surgically removed at that time. He had more recently lost over one-tenth of his body weight and was very weak. He admitted that he had been suffering from sharp pains in the rectum and constipation, but he had had two X-rays and an ultrasound scan in the previous month, all of which had showed nothing wrong in the lower bowel and rectum.

At the end of the consultation I said I would do a report of the findings immediately and send it to his naturopath, but I suggested he ask his surgeon to do a more thorough rectal examination on his next visit to the hospital. It transpired that his next appointment with the surgeon treating his cancer was the following day; Mr R explained that the pains in his backside were getting worse, so to pacify him, and to investigate further, the surgeon carried out a colonoscopy, which revealed a malignant growth a little way up the rectum.

Mr R's wife came to see me by herself some time later, and she told me that the surgeon had informed her six months previously that her husband's cancer had spread into the lymphatic system (hence the brightness of the arcus senilis). Mr R fought his condition with allopathic and alternative medicine, but the problem had progressed too far, and several months later he died. He was one of the bravest and most courageous men I have been honoured to meet.

12
HOW TO ANALYSE AN IRIS

Now that we have covered the theory behind iris analysis, we can begin to put some of it into practice. By this stage you should have an idea as to what part of the iris relates to what part of the body, and what the various colours and markings indicate in relation to the state of health. So it is now simply a matter of putting together all the basic principles set out in the preceding chapters in order to begin a health analysis based on an investigation of the irises.

THE TOOLS

There is very little required in the way of utensils in order to analyse an iris. All we really need is a magnifying lens (with preferably a minimum of 10X magnification), a pen-light, and a pencil and notepad to record the markings. There are several other gadgets available that have a light-powered source and magnifying lens combined, the most popular of which is a Peak Light Loupe; however, although this enables one hand to be kept free, most people find that a simple magnifying lens and pen-light are easier to use.

Camera Equipment

In my practice I use a video-iriscope, a machine I developed with the help of an optometrist from optical photographic equipment. It magnifies the iris by up to 80 times and then transmits the image on to a monitor, from where it is stored on video-tape. This type of equipment, and other specialised cameras, provide greater detail of an iris, and enable exact records to be taken so that an iris can be analysed at leisure rather than having to have the person sitting in front of you. However, the main advantage is that a patient can see their own irises and the various conditions can be pointed out; photographs and video film of a patient's eyes thus give the patient a better understanding of what the practitioner is talking about.

SELF ANALYSIS

It is not difficult to analyse one's own irises. The same procedure is adopted as for examining someone else's irises, although it is easier to use a contactoscope to look at one's own eyes. A contactoscope is a small battery-operated machine made up of a small concave mirror with 10× magnification and an internal light source. It was developed for contact lens users to check on their contact lenses, but it works just as well for a self iris analysis.

When looking at one's own eyes, remember that, as in all mirror images, the chart must be turned around. Another point to consider when attempting to do a self analysis is that it is extremely difficult to remain dispassionate and objective; however, as long as you record exactly what you see, you will have a fairly accurate analysis.

TECHNIQUE FOR ANALYSING AN IRIS

When examining a person's irises there are a few things to consider. For instance, try not to keep the light shining on the eye for more than 10 to 15 seconds at a time, as longer periods may irritate the eye's delicate membranes. Quickly examine the iris, make a few notes and then, after giving the eye a rest from the light, repeat the procedure until the analysis is complete.

Whenever I use a magnifying lens and pen-light, I find it is easiest and most comfortable when examining someone's right iris to hold the magnifying glass in my right hand under the person's right eye, and the pen-light in my left hand, held 4–5 inches away from the person's face and with the light being directed from the side. This way is much more comfortable and less tiring for the patient than having a light shining straight on the eye.

Finally, it goes without saying that it is not advisable to sit too close to the patient, breathing all over him or her, especially if, for example, you recently ate garlic!

The procedure for analysing an iris is best kept simple and methodical. This way it can be completed quickly and efficiently. Most practitioners develop their own style and sequence, but I usually start by examining the right iris and then go on to the left, using the four stages of analysis set out below:

- Mark down the base colour of the iris, and note any apparent discolourations and then locations.
- Mark down the iris structure, again noting any deviations and their locations.
- Go through the main body systems, one by one, noting the specific iris signs.
- Finally, note the general constitution, i.e. the iris constitution that most closely resembles the iris under examination, and then any other iris constitutions that may relate to the iris in question.

In the accompanying box is a simple structured form that goes through this method of iris analysis.

Remember, whatever you may find, there is never any need to worry. There is very little that the body cannot heal. This is not a time for despondency, it is a time for excitement. It is a turning point in your life; a time to change for the better, for creating a brighter future. It provides the basis for designing a remedial and preventive health programme to improve the state of your health and the quality of your life. And if there is anything that you are at all concerned about, don't panic! Simply make an appointment to see an iridologist in your locality.

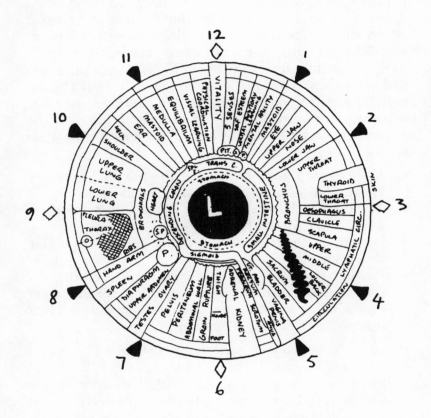

THE IRIS MAP – LEFT EYE
(mirror image of one's own left eye)

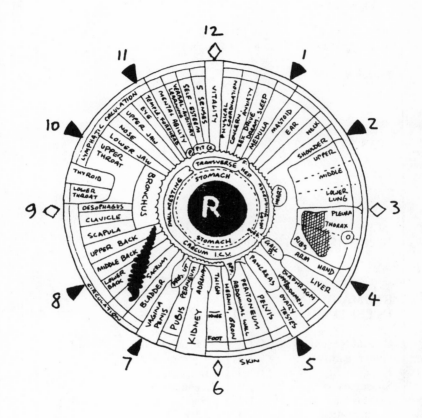

THE IRIS MAP – RIGHT EYE
(mirror image of one's own right eye)

IRIS ANALYSIS FORM

NAME   DATE

IRIS COLOUR   Blue [ ]   Brown [ ]   Mixed [ ]

Comments

IRIS STRUCTURE   Silk [ ]   Linen [ ]   Hessian [ ]   Net [ ]

Comments

GENERAL CONSTITUTION

STOMACH AND INTESTINES	R	L	**NERVOUS**	R	L
Central toxaemia	[ ]	[ ]	Tension rings	[ ]	[ ]
Hyper-acidity	[ ]	[ ]	Tight pupil	[ ]	[ ]
Hypo-acidity	[ ]	[ ]	Large pupil	[ ]	[ ]
Spastic colon	[ ]	[ ]	Head acute	[ ]	[ ]
Tight colon	[ ]	[ ]	Head chronic	[ ]	[ ]
Inflammation	[ ]	[ ]	ANW	[ ]	[ ]
Impactions	[ ]	[ ]	Pupil distortion	[ ]	[ ]

Comments   Comments

CARDIO-VASCULAR	R	L	**RESPIRATORY**	R	L
Scurf rim	[ ]	[ ]	Strong tissue	[ ]	[ ]
Arcus senilis	[ ]	[ ]	Weak tissue	[ ]	[ ]

Heart (weak)	[ ] [ ]	Congestion (lung)	[ ] [ ]
Poor circulation	[ ] [ ]	Congestion (bronchial)	[ ] [ ]
Tendency v.veins	[ ] [ ]	Congestion (throat)	[ ] [ ]

Comments   Comments

LYMPHATIC	**R**	**L**	**URINARY/ REPRODUCTIVE**	**R**	**L**
Congestion	[ ]	[ ]	Kidneys, weak	[ ]	[ ]
Lymphatic Rosary	[ ]	[ ]	Kidneys, congestion	[ ]	[ ]
			Bladder	[ ]	[ ]
			Prostate/uterus	[ ]	[ ]
			Penis/vagina	[ ]	[ ]

Comments   Comments

MUSCULAR/ SKELETAL	**R**	**L**	**MISCELLANEOUS**	**R**	**L**
Inflammation	[ ]	[ ]	Liver	[ ]	[ ]
Loose tissue	[ ]	[ ]	Gall bladder	[ ]	[ ]
Transverse fibres	[ ]	[ ]	Pancreas	[ ]	[ ]
Neck/shoulder	[ ]	[ ]	Thyroid	[ ]	[ ]
Arm	[ ]	[ ]	Pituitary	[ ]	[ ]
Spine	[ ]	[ ]	Spleen	[ ]	[ ]
Leg	[ ]	[ ]			

Comments   Comments

GENERAL COMMENTS

FINDING AND VISITING A PRACTITIONER

By far the best way of contacting a reputable iridologist is through personal recommendation or, failing that, by writing one of the addresses listed on page 270. Consultation fees tend to range dramatically depending upon the location of the clinic, the equipment used by the clinic, the length of time required by the practitioner, and any other facilities offered by the clinic.

Most iridologists practise other forms of complementary medicine, whether it be homoeopathy, osteopathy, naturopathy, herbalism, or nutrition. It is therefore advisable to telephone first and ask the practitioner about his or her practice, and particularly his or her treatments. There are many ways to crack a nut, and the treatments offered by a practitioner will depend upon his or her training and those therapies with which he or she has most confidence and experience. This may or may not be to your liking, so it is therefore important to establish that you are happy with the practitioner's mode of treatments before you make the appointment.

The first consultation will normally last about an hour, but some practitioners somehow manage to do it within 15 minutes, whereas others can take up to two hours. In this time the practitioner will examine your irises, and ask you about your symptoms, illnesses, family and medical history and your general lifestyle. It will save time and help the practitioner if, before you go, you have notes ready on all the medicines and supplements you may currently be taking, as well as details of your family and medical history and the symptoms, if any, that you are experiencing.

It is from the iris analysis and other information gleaned from this initial appointment that a remedial or preventive programme can be drawn up to deal with the conditions seen in the eye. This may involve specific treatments (e.g. a course of acupuncture, reflexology or homoeopathy) or it may include naturopathic home treatments, herbal remedies and dietary guidelines of a similar nature to those mentioned in this book. My personal belief is that all treatments are a substitute for correct living habits, and it is therefore far preferable to balance one's lifestyle than take tablets of any kind (whether herbal, homoeopathic or allopathic). True health is created only by healthy living.

THE DIFFERENT SCHOOLS OF IRIDOLOGY

There are many different schools and various approaches to the study and practice of iridology. One of the most remarkable features of the history of iris diagnosis is the fact that its discovery came about in various countries through the work of different people, and yet all came to very similar conclusions. Despite this, iridologists from the various countries, using empirical research and clinical observation, have developed their own very distinct approaches to the science, with different emphases on interpretations and different remedial treatments.

The Germans for instance take a purely physical diagnosis, whereas in America the Rayid school concentrates solely on a psychological interpretation. Not surprisingly, the suggested treatment is on a physical level in Germany, while the Rayid school advise an emotional/psychological approach to remedial treatment. The two schools are thus as different as chalk and cheese, and yet both are of value in holistic and preventive medicine, where it has long been acknowledged that the mind and body are not mutually exclusive but completely interdependent.

Europe was the birthplace of modern iridology, and much of the early progress was made in Germany, where medical practitioners began considering how the various markings in the iris related to the disorders suffered by the patients. But whilst the early German iridologists wrote of psychological disturbances recorded in the iris, they did not delve very far into this aspect and instead chose to concentrate on the physiological findings. Ultimately the late Joseph Deck came to the point whereby he was able to categorise the different types of iris into 'constitutional' types, treatment first being prescribed according to the constitution and only later for any specific disorders. I had the opportunity of studying at the International Institute of Iris Diagnosis in Ettlingen, Germany, which was founded by Joseph Deck and which concentrates on treatments using a variety of homoeopathic medications and preparations.

The Jensen school in the USA also places emphasis on the physiological findings in the iris. As Jensen is a manipulative therapist and naturopath, treatments are also on a physical level, using mineral supplements, dietary guidelines, naturopathic remedies and, of course, manipulative treatments. However Jensen did not rule out the effect of the mind on the body, and his chart included areas at the top of the iris which related to psychological and emotional conditions. Just as the mind affects the body, so does the body affect the mind; so it is that the physical treatments are emphasised, particularly the cleansing of the colon, in order to deal with both physical and psychological disorders.

Denny Johnson, founder of the Rayid method of iris interpretation was more interested in whether different character traits and personality types were revealed in the iris, and particularly whether they could be categorised into different iris types. The Rayid method thus concentrates solely on the emotional/psychological factors and how these affect the iris, and is of great value in establishing mental cause for physical ailments but not vice versa.

Dorothy Hall is probably the most notable of present-day Australian iridologists, and she uses a more pragmatic approach, taking into account both mind and body. Perhaps the most important contribution to the science of iridology made by Ms Hall was her challenge to the early iridologists' claim that there are perfect and imperfect irises, the perfect being clear blue or brown with closely knit fibres and no discolourations, and the imperfect being anything else. The Australian school takes the view that, whilst the clear iris with closely knit tissue resembling silk may be physiologically strong, it is neurogenically weaker, as the silk-type person generally has excess nervous energy and is less sensitive to his own needs and the needs of those about him than other iris types. In contrast, the iris with loosely knit fibres resembling a net, although physically weaker than the silk iris, is emotionally stronger and more able to filter out unwanted or negative emotions.

In all its various approaches, iridology has a lot to offer in the treatment of all disorders, and especially in preventive health care, because without an accurate health analysis or diagnosis all treatment is guesswork. Iridology shows constitutional strengths and weaknesses and the state of each organ in the body. One remarkable feature of iris diagnosis is the fact that changes appear in the iris prior to the physical symptom, and therefore preventive action can be taken to avoid those diseases that might otherwise ensue. For instance, where it is seen that there is weak tissue in the kidney area of the iris, the patient should avoid those foods and substances that put unnecessary strain on the kidneys, and perhaps take a herbal remedy to strengthen the kidneys. Where there is toxicity in the alimentary tract, again changes can be made to the patient's lifestyle to prevent future problems with the digestive tract. Pinpointing weaknesses and danger spots can alert the patient so that preventive measures can be taken.

PART II
DESIGNING YOUR PREVENTIVE HEALTH CARE PROGRAMME

It cannot be denied that it is the physician as 'preventer of ills' who will be the doctor of the future . . . preventive medicine will be the supreme human science of this century.

Sir W. Arbuthnot Lane, British surgeon, 1934

The doctor of the future will give no medicine but will interest his patients in the care of the human frame, in diet, and in the cause and prevention of disease.

Thomas Edison

13
PREVENTIVE
HEALTH CARE

Now there were some terrible seeds on the planet that was the home of the little prince; and these were the seeds of the baobab. The soil of that planet was infested with them. A baobab is something you will never, never be able to get rid of if you attend to it too late. It spreads over the entire planet. It bores clear through with its roots. And if the planet is too small and the baobabs too many, they split it into may pieces . . .

You must see to it that you pull up regularly all the baobabs, at the very first moment when they can be distinguished from the rose bushes . . . there is no harm putting off a piece of work until another day. But when it is a matter of baobabs, that always means catastrophe.

Antoine de Saint-Exupéry,   *The Little Prince*

Preventive health care is about dealing with conditions before they manifest themselves in a disease or disorder; it is about maintaining health rather than dealing with disease. The World Health Organisation has stated that at least 85 per cent of all diseases are preventable. Yet today the number of deaths due to heart and circulatory diseases and cancer continues to rise. The frequency of diabetes mellitus is increasing rapidly, and the potential for children to become diabetic is significantly greater than for their parents.

In fact all chronic degenerative diseases are increasing at alarming rates, mainly because we refuse to acknowledge a simple law of health and disease, the law of cause and effect. We reap only that which we have sown. It is the things we do in life – our food, our posture, our emotions, our exercise – that create either health or disease. For every symptom or illness we suffer, there is a cause, and until we are willing to respect this law, the best we can do is mask over the symptoms. But we will never find true health.

Preventive health is thus a simple three-step procedure:

- Look to the law of cause and effect.
- Eliminate the cause.
- Create the conditions within the body for an active healing force.

THE LAW OF CAUSE AND EFFECT

The law of cause and effect operates throughout life. Nothing occurs out of nothing. Just as the law of gravity dictates that an apple dropped from the top of a building will fall to the ground, so too does the law of cause and effect dictate that for every symptom or illness we may suffer there will always be a cause.

Imagine for a moment you are hammering a picture-nail into the wall and suddenly you miss the nail and hit your thumb. You wash your thumb, put some ointment on, and bandage it. Five minutes later you go back to the hammering, and once again hit your thumb. What chance do you think there will be that your thumb will heal whilst you continue hammering away, hitting it with a hammer? Painkillers may eliminate the pain, and anti-inflammatory medications may reduce the inflammation, but the thumb will never get better whilst you continue to hit it.

The same law applies for injuries inside the body. A stomach ulcer will never heal until the cause of the hyperacidity, whether it be a high level of acid-forming foods in the diet and/or emotional stress, can be found and eliminated. Anti-acid tablets may suppress the symptoms and alleviate the pain, but they will not cure the condition. If you do not deal with the cause of the condition, the condition will only worsen. There is only one way to heal the ulcer and ensure it does not return – find and eliminate the cause. Were you eating acid-forming foods? Had you been under a lot of stress, which itself can cause acidity? If so, do something about it.

Treating a symptom, whether it be a neck ache, a skin complaint, a stomach ulcer, a nervous disorder or a cancerous growth, with a chemical never leads to health. All chemical tablets, lotions, creams and powders at best may alleviate the pain. At worse they cause a plethora of side effects, so that at the end of the treatment the underlying condition will have worsened, simply because the cause of the problem is still there, the hammer is still banging away.

But once you eliminate the cause, once you stop hitting your thumb, the body's healing force will spring into action, and the thumb will heal itself – without any tablets, potions, lotions or creams. The thumb will heal because we all have a healing force within us.

THE ACTIVE HEALING FORCE

The body has its own defence mechanism, its healing powers are kept at work in the body, powers from which our therapeutics are a very long distance behind.

Dr Richard C. Cabot

There is a life force that pervades nature, a force given to each and every one of us from birth by nature to keep us healthy and to heal us in times of distress.

However, the healing force is often damaged or destroyed by our own doing. For instance, part of the healing force consists of the white blood cells (leucocytes) that travel through the bloodstream destroying invading bacteria. But many people make themselves and their children more open to infections and diseases simply by eating excess sugar. It has been shown in clinical tests that the consumption of six teaspoons of white sugar in one day will reduce the number of leucocytes within the body by approximatgely 25 per cent, and this reduction in white blood cells will worsen in increasing proportions with the more sugar consumed. Six teaspoons of sugar are all that is needed, and these are often hidden in cookies, chocolates, cakes, tinned food and fruit yoghurts, to name but a few; a typical fruit yoghurt, for instance, contains three teaspoons of sugar, and some chocolate bars contain over 12 teaspoons of sugar. So we can begin to see how those few teaspoons of sugar in cups of coffee and the daily chocolate bar may, in the long term, have catastrophic consequences for our healing force and thus our state of health.

In order to be healthy we must therefore avoid those things that destroy the healing force and do those things that encourage a strong and active healing or life force within the body.

MAINTAINING HEALTH

An iceberg is not just the tip that we can see lying above the surface of the water; it also has an enormous mass lying deep below the ocean. Similarly, disease is not just the symptoms we feel; it is the condition of the tissue inside the body, that we cannot see. Many diseases are slow insidious processes, and the symptoms are the last things to occur in that process.

The water level on the iceberg thus represents the symptom level; it is the point at which we feel the pain, and therefore it is also the point at which we seek help. Suppressive medications merely act to raise the water level nearer the very tip of the iceberg, the tip in this case representing the point at which the condition becomes terminal, the point of no return. In preventive health care we are thus concerned with maintaining a state of health that is normally concealed well below the surface level of the water.

The practical difficulty of maintaining health lies only with our attitude towards our health, and our priorities in life. Most people say that they want health and happiness, but they do not want to do the things that are necessary to create health and happiness. Indeed, many people do not want to make even the most basic changes in their lifestyle for the sake of their health; for example, they are simply not prepared to stop smoking, to change their diet, or to take up regular exercise. After all, they say, isn't it so much easier to take a tablet?

It is true that sticking to a natural wholesome diet at first takes effort and discipline, as it often conflicts with family traditions, social functions, even business luncheons – and it is just as often these family traditions, social engagements and business meetings that are considered more important than the individual's health. Doing daily exercises, finding time to relax and confronting deep-rooted emotional resentment all require time set aside during the day; but, again, most individuals will only do these if there is time to spare after they have done everything else.

So, whilst most people will, when asked, say that health is their number one priority in life, it soon becomes clear that health often doesn't even come close to the top of a person's list of priorities. But in preventive health care we must follow nature's laws, and in many cases this means that fundamental changes must be made in our lives.

THE ONE-DEGREE PRINCIPLE

Every minute of every day we are changing. We are changing physically, as every minute of every day thousands upon thousands of body cells are dying off and being replaced by new ones; in effect, within the space of a few weeks, we are completely different physical structures to what we had been.

But we are also changing emotionally, mentally and even spiritually as, day by day, we live new experiences and learn new lessons that help change our emotional states and spiritual outlook. Changes of foods we eat, changes of moods, new experiences, all affect our health.

So why not consciously make positive changes? Radical

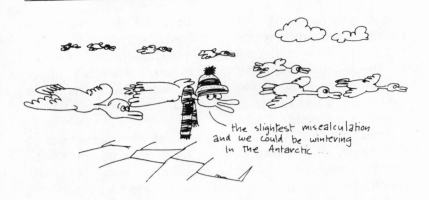

the slightest miscalculation and we could be wintering in the Antarctic ...

changes are not necessary in order to begin to notice how you can improve your health. Imagine a bird migrating from England to Africa in the winter; if it changes its course by only one or two degrees it may eventually end up in India instead. Similarly, life can be likened to a journey, and small changes in the course of our direction will in the long term lead us to a completely different destination. Imagine that you are walking in a straight line, and this line represents where you are going in life. If you make a small alteration in your direction by only one degree, within the space of a few hundred metres you would soon find that you are in a completely different place from where you would have been had you stayed on the original course. In the same way, it does not require big changes or alterations in lifestyle to create big changes in an individual's health.

This is the one-degree principle – the smallest change can produce a big impact on your health in the long term. Preventive health is not about instant radical change. It is about small, slow changes in lifestyle which will positively affect our health and well-being.

PAIN – FRIEND OR FOE?

Pain is the one thing we try to avoid at all cost. Everything in life we do is motivated by our desire to attain pleasure or to avoid pain. Nobody likes pain, and why should they?

It hurts! But did you ever stop to consider what would happen if we did not feel any pain?

You might be sitting next to a fire, and a few minutes later notice that your arm had been burned. Pain is thus not an enemy; it is a friend, telling you that something has gone wrong and that you should do something about it.

Most people try to eliminate pain as quickly as possible with strong medications. The drug companies were quick to see that a person will pay a high price to get rid of pain. Every year new and improved painkilling drugs come on to the market, most of which get taken off again because of the toxic side effects, leaving the patient not only with the original problem but also with the added burden of having to deal with the side effects of the medications.

I recall seeing one man who had suffered for years with migraine. His doctor had prescribed a medicine which didn't affect his migraine but which did raise his blood pressure to an unacceptably high level. As a result he had to have further tablets to lower the blood pressure. Eventually he began to change his lifestyle by taking regular exercise and adopting a healthier diet, avoiding known migraine irritants such as chocolate, hard cheeses, red meats and alcohol. Within a few months his migraine attacks had been dramatically reduced from five a week to two a month, and the attacks subsequently became fewer and fewer over the following year. He then went back to his doctor to tell him of the good news and to confirm that he no longer needed to stay on the medication. It was then the doctor dropped the bombshell – the man would have to stay on blood pressure tablets for the rest of his life.

Pain is for your benefit. It is nature's voice. We can either listen to it or close our ears, but if you kill pain, you are on the way to killing yourself.

DRUGS AND DISEASE

Drugs never cure disease in the body. It may be true that antibiotics will kill strains of invading bacteria, but as mentioned earlier, the bacteria are not the disease. The dis-ease is actually the under-functioning immune system.

In fact, rather than 'cure' disease, it has now become widely recognised that drugs actually *cause* disease. Medical historian Ivan Illich, on the first page of his book *Medical Nemesis*, predicted 'Modern medicine will become the biggest threat to public health'. Today that prediction has come true, with by far and away the biggest cause of hospital admissions being from the side effects of drugs; studies have shown that somewhere between one-quarter and one-third of all hospital patients are admitted as a direct result of the drugs they were given.

Every year over 15,000 new medications come on to the market, but approximately 12,000 get withdrawn because of toxic side effects (and many of those end up being dumped on Third World populations, where government regulations are more relaxed concerning unsafe medications). There are over 350,000 different drugs available, yet the World Health Organisation has categorically stated that only 26 are 'necessary' for health (which implies that all the others are unnecessary), while a UNESCO committee concluded that of those 26 only nine were 'absolutely essential' (again implying that all of the others are not absolutely essential). At the top of that list was aspirin, but even that was later found to cause gastrointestinal bleeding in over three-quarters of the people who regularly took it, and liver and brain damage when given to children.

Drugs are often an easy way out in the short term, but in the long term they spell disaster.

THE TIME FOR CHANGE AND ACTION

There is a saying in North America that most people change only when they are sick and tired of being sick and tired. Preventive medicine is about dealing with the baobabs inside our bodies; it is about intelligent change, before disease catches up with us; it is about changing without being sick, and without being tired of being sick and tired. It is about living with health as your number

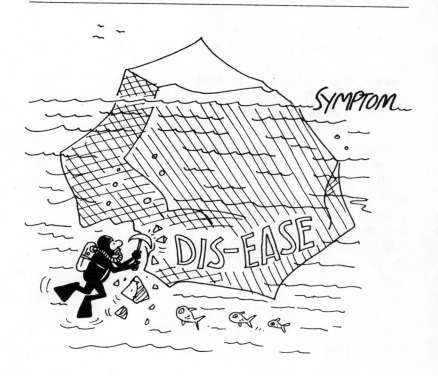

one priority, because when you are healthy your quality of life soars. It is about breaking up the iceberg, piece by piece, all the way down to its very foundations.

The secret of health lies in prevention, not cure. It is not just because of the futility of closing the stable door after the horse has bolted, but because there is no cure other than the body's own healing force, and creating an active healing force is our own responsibility. No tablet, whether allopathic, homoeopathic or herbal, will cure your body. The only cure comes from the body's natural healing force. When you cut yourself the body stops the loss of blood with a blood clot, and increases the numbers of white blood cells in order to fight any infection. If we work with nature we can assist the healing by washing and bandaging the wound, but nothing that we do will cure it.

Therefore, to prevent chronic disease and maintain health we must possess an active healing force within us,

139

and this can only be achieved through our lifestyle – diet, posture, exercise, emotional and physical stress – in sum, how we live.

And where does iris analysis fit into this? With iris analysis we can see the baobabs; we can see the iceberg below the water; we can lock the stable door whilst the horse remains inside; we can have 20/20 vision without hindsight. Iris analysis offers the basis for a healthier future by indicating areas where a preventive and remedial health care programme can be applied to assist the body's own healing force naturally.

Baobabs don't just grow on the little prince's planet; they flourish here on Earth, and they even grow inside our bodies, albeit that doctors have given them new names. Carcinomas, viruses and bacteria are all of the same family as the baobab, because if they are not rooted out at the earliest opportunity they spread over the entire body and slowly destroy it. Therefore we must learn to respect the baobab for what it is, and diligently dig it up wherever it may be found.

14
DESIGNING A PREVENTIVE HEALTH CARE PROGRAMME

To be what we are and to become what we are capable of becoming is the only creed in life.

Robert Louis Stevenson

Once you know where you are and where you want to go, nothing, but nothing, can stop you getting there. In Part I of this book you were told about the tools that iris analysis gives you, whereby you can use your eyes to find out about yourself, your physical and emotional make-up. The simple techniques of iris analysis will indicate the condition of the organs and tissues in your body, and will point to the likely causes of your present condition.

But knowledge by itself is useless, and remains so unless and until it can be applied in our daily lives. This part of the book is about putting that knowledge into action; it is about taking that first step along a new path to health; it is about drawing up and adopting a preventive health programme.

The preventive health programme is an initial three-month programme specifically designed to deal with the conditions found in your iris analysis, rather than aimed at simply treating any symptoms from which you might be suffering. (But do remember, if you are taking any medications for any conditions, or you are under the care or supervision of your doctor or hospital, please ensure that you seek their advice and approval before embarking on any health programme.) The programme aims to deal naturally with the underlying causes of any health problems, helping to create the conditions within the body for the body to heal itself and thereafter to maintain a high level of health. It involves dietary guidelines suited to your constitution, herbal fluid extracts, tissue salts and other naturopathic treatments, all aimed at strengthening any weaknesses located by iris analysis and at building on your strengths. Remember, health is created only by healthy living. There is no magic potion or tablet; it is simply a question of lifestyle and adhering as best you can to the laws of health. Just as the law of gravity dictates that an apple on a tree will fall to the ground, so do the laws of health dictate that health can be achieved only by looking after three main aspects of health:

- Diet.
- Physical health.
- Emotional/spiritual health.

And all three aspects need to be considered in any health programme.

In order to make it through any programme or regimen, right from the outset there are three steps necessary to ensure success.

- Notice.
- Take action.
- Notice your outcome and take further action.

NOTICE

Before starting any journey it is always prudent to take notice – notice where you are and where you want to go, notice the things about you that will slow you down and notice those things that may help you. Noticing is essential to going anywhere or doing anything with your life.

So, before embarking on the preventive health care programme, stop for a moment and notice how you feel, and how you would like to feel. In terms of health, you must ask yourself what you want, what you believe you can achieve, and how much of your existing lifestyle you are willing to sacrifice in order to achieve it.

If the state of your health could be measured on a scale from 1 to 10, 1 meaning that you are dead and 10 meaning that you feel on top of the world, what number would most accurately reflect your health at the moment? Asking yourself this question may be the first time that you have really considered your present state of health and, more importantly, what improvement you believe is possible. But, it is an important question to reflect upon as it helps us consider our potential in health and how much more we may be able to get out of life.

What number represents your level of health? How much of an improvement do you believe you can make?

The importance of having a goal

A goal is something to aim for, something to strive towards, and something that creates commitment. Goals put purpose and meaning into our actions.

Most of us do not live up to even a fraction of our potential. What we are is far far less than what we could be. This is partly because we sometimes impose our own limitations on ourselves; we believe it's normal to have aching joints in middle age, or it's normal to have arthritis; it's normal to be tired or to have high cholesterol levels in the blood when you reach the age of 50. While these problems may all be common, they are certainly not normal. In fact all of these beliefs are nonsense. The only thing that is 'normal' or 'natural' as far as the human body is concerned is a state of health. Any dis-ease and dis-order is unnatural and abnormal.

The truth is that we impose our own limitations on our lives. We can be what we want to be and become what we want to become. Of course, a man of 50 years is not likely to grow another foot taller (although by improving his posture he may gain a few inches) and likewise the size of a woman's nose is unlikely to change considerably. But, as

143

far as health is concerned, there are very few limitations. If there is one saying that has helped people to see a better future it is that given by Anthony Robbins in his bestselling book *Unlimited Power*: 'The past does not equal the future'.

Just because yesterday you may have had indigestion, or migraine, or a skin complaint, or anything else you care to mention, that does not mean that you will have it tomorrow. It is only if you do what you have always done that you will get what you have always got.

So why not set new goals, new standards and new challenges? Imagine yourself the way you want to be, and write down on a piece of paper a full description of how you see yourself, physically and emotionally. Write down the activities you will be doing, the feelings you will be feeling. Write it all down and keep that piece of paper in a safe place. Now you have an outcome, a goal to aim for.

Decide to succeed

Decide right from the beginning that, come what may, you will follow the programme through to the end. It is not sufficient to decide to try it for a while and see how it goes. Commit yourself to the programme. Your health is literally in your hands. Your health can improve or worsen; you have the power to build it or destroy it, and you can start building or demolishing today.

ACTION

> If one advances confidently in the direction of his dreams, and endeavors to live the live which he has imagined, he will meet with a success unexpected in common hours.
>
> Henry David Thoreau

Power is defined by the *Concise Oxford Dictionary* as 'the ability to do something'; in other words the ability to act is power. Therefore we all have personal power. But some people choose not to use it; they choose not to take action. Yet it is action that separates those people who succeed in life from those who do not.

Education, family background, money, good looks, friends in the right places may all be of value, but the essential ingredient to ensure success, whether in following a health programme or finding a job, is action. For action is power. Action is the difference between reality and dreams; it is the major difference between those who achieve their goals and those who don't. Without taking action nothing gets done and nothing is achieved. All the knowledge and information on healthy living in the world is useless unless it is acted upon. Having an intention to do something is not enough. It is necessary to take control and do it; whether it be sticking to dietary guidelines or taking up daily exercise, it must be acted upon for you to derive any benefit.

Without taking that first step, we are no closer to our desired destination. However, once we take one step, the next step follows more easily. Therefore start off the way you mean to continue, and take action. This is essentially what the preventive health care programme is; a plan of action to move you towards a healthier life.

CONTINUING TO TAKE ACTION

There will be times when we go off course, but we all need to do this occasionally. Indeed, there are no straight lines in life, only ups and downs, or peaks and troughs. A straight line indicates stagnation and, in some circumstances, death. Imagine a heart rate monitor; the trace goes up and down until the heart stops, at which point it becomes a straight line.

So there will be times when you notice that you have gone off course – a sudden seemingly uncontrollable urge to assault a family pack of double-creamed double-layered chocolate cookies, or the need to sneak a few puffs of a cigarette. But don't use these times as an excuse to quit the programme. Simply recommit yourself to the programme, and take the requisite action to get back on course.

This is exactly what every pilot does every time he makes a flight. In fact during any flight the airplane will be off course approximately 95 per cent of the time, due to changes in altitude, wind, turbulence and other climatic conditions. But as soon as the pilot notices that he is off course he takes further action to get back on target and, apart from exceptional circumstances, he always reaches his desired destination.

DESIGNING YOUR PLAN OF ACTION

The first stage in designing your programme is to complete your iris analysis. Then simply refer to the relevant sections in this part of the book to find out the suggested preventive measures for the condition or conditions that have been revealed by the analysis. For example, if you have found that you have an arcus senilis, go to the chapter on the cardiovascular system and look for the section referring to arcus senilis.

Once you have referred to all the conditions in your iris health screen form (pages 122–3), you will then have a complete health care programme. However, don't try to take on board the whole programme at once; it could prove extremely difficult, and may even overwhelm you. Instead, it is much easier to do it one step at a time.

For instance, sort out the dietary guidelines during the first week, the herbal remedies in the second week, and the other recommendations in the following weeks. Adopt the one-degree principle and take it a little at a time. This way you will find the programme easy to follow and you will make great progress.

The reason why so many people get better once they have adopted their health care programme is that there is no guesswork. You no longer have to try a vitamin, mineral tablet or potion and hope for the best. Now, you know what to do. The programme simply respects the laws of health. For every cause there is an effect; if you remove the cause, you will remove the effect.

One *caveat*. Nature works, but it works slowly. This is the reason why the programme must be continued for a minimum of three months. Most people will feel substantial improvement during that time. However, just as some conditions take a long time to surface, so they will also take a long time to go away.

Please also remember that the basic law of cure, as stated by the 19th-century homoeopath, Constantine Hering, is that:

Cure takes place from above downward, from within outward, from an important organ to a less important organ; symptoms disappear in reverse order of their appearance, the first thing to appear being the last to disappear.

Thus every symptom that occurred as the dis-ease progressed will also re-occur as the dis-ease regresses, and in the reverse order. For example, if someone suffered from migraines and then stomach pains followed by nausea, during the healing process they might experience nausea followed by stomach cramps and then migraines. The iris markings will also change as and when the healing process progresses, and these you will be able to monitor.

The programme is gentle, and designed to minimise such cleansing reactions, but should you re-experience old symptoms, don't panic. They should last only a few days. Do not use any suppressive medications (unless so prescribed by your doctor), and the symptoms will go within a few days. But if you have any doubts at all please consult your health practitioner.

Finally, may I stress again how important it is to be committed to your goal of a healthier life. All change takes effort, but in the end it pays high dividends in the improved quality of life. Your health is in your hands – you have the power to take control of and responsibility for your own health. This programme may mark the beginning of a new direction in your life; may you be blessed with health and happiness along the way.

15
THE RESPIRATORY SYSTEM

And the Lord ... breathed into his nostrils the breath of life, and man became a living soul.

Genesis 2,7

Breathing is the most natural and vital of functions, an instinct which many of us lose over the years as we go about our sedentary jobs, cooped up in air-conditioned offices and doing little or no exercise. Slowly we become shallow breathers, the diaphragm sags and stale air accumulates in the lungs. The body is then poorly oxygenated, we become sluggish, and mucus congestion develops, not just in the respiratory tract but throughout the entire body. And if that wasn't enough to cope with, the art of efficient breathing has been further hindered by our constant exposure to the mass of traffic and industrial waste fumes.

When one is born with strong tissue in the lungs and bronchials, the damage can be put off for some time. But when the tissue is inherently weak, problems develop sooner rather than later – asthma, hayfever, bronchitis, pneumonia, emphysema, and a host of other complaints. Nothing happens by chance, and the only way to keep the respiratory system healthy is to take preventive measures in order to strengthen our weaknesses.

WEAK LUNG TISSUE

Where the lung tissue is weak you should immediately stop smoking, and avoid mucus-forming foods (e.g. dairy foods, red meats, refined white flour and white sugar foods), as weak tissue cannot throw off congestion efficiently.

Deep inhalations using olbas oil in boiling water and deep breathing exercises are particularly helpful in stimulating the lungs and bronchial tubes to throw out mucus congestion.

Deep breathing

There are two particular deep breathing exercises that are excellent for strengthening the lung tissues and increasing your lung capacity.

Whilst walking Deep breathing exercises can be performed easily whilst walking in the park, countryside or by the roadside (however don't bother where there is a lot of traffic congestion as you will merely inhale more fumes).

- Inhale for the count of, say, 4 paces.
- Hold for the count of 4 paces.
- Exhale for the count of 8 paces.
- Hold again for the count of 4 paces.
- Keep to the same ratio (inhale 1: hold 1: exhale 2: hold 1), and try to build it up to 7 paces for inhalation.

Whilst relaxing When sitting or lying down you can do the following exercises. It will help you to relax for a few minutes, and afterwards you will feel the energising effects. The exercise can be done anywhere – in the office, park, etc. – but again not where there are heavy fumes. When you do the exercise, try to breathe from the stomach, using your diaphragm, rather than the 'top' of chest.

The cycle is best done in repetitions of 10, three times each day as follows:

- Inhale 7 seconds.
- Hold 28 seconds.
- Exhale 14 seconds.

If you cannot manage 7 seconds, do the exercise for a shorter period, but keep the same ratio, i.e. inhale 1: hold 4: exhale 2.

The benefits – and a warning   The reason for holding the inhalation for four units of time during the resting exercise and only one unit when walking is that holding the breath in for a prolonged period of time during exercise can create too much strain.

These exercises will slowly build up your lung capacity and help cleanse the lymphatic system. In time you will instinctively breathe more and more deeply. However, they are certainly not as easy as they sound, so please remember not to strain or create stress; simply build up slowly and comfortably to the recommended levels.

CONGESTED LUNGS

Where there is congestion in the lungs, the same treatment as above should be carried out. However, you should expect to have one or two colds as a result, because at some stage the mucus congestion will have to be eliminated, and there is only one way for it to come out.

It is also important to sleep with the window open, even in cold weather, to allow fresh air to circulate at night. Most people work all day in a stagnant environment, with so-called 'air-conditioning' (recycled stale air), and then go home to sleep in rooms that are poorly ventilated. This is a sure recipe for disaster in the long term, and the respirattory system can only deteriorate under such a regimen.

CONGESTION IN THE UPPER BRONCHUS, THROAT AND SINUSES

Where the upper bronchus and throat are congested, an old yogic method of morning throat cleansing can be performed on a daily basis (for a minimum period of 10 days).

- The night before mix the juice of half a lemon and a teaspoon of honey in a glass of water. Then in the morning:
- Scrape the mucus off the back of the tongue with an inverted spoon.
- Inhale cold water 10 times up each nostril until the water can be felt on the back of the throat, and then blow your nose.
- Gargle with the lemon and honey water.

The onion and honey remedy

In acute cases of congestion in the throat try the onion and honey cure. Pour half a pound of acacia honey on top of raw chopped-up onion, and leave overnight; it will turn into a runny juice by the morning. Sip a teaspoon of the juice regularly at half hourly intervals.

Onion has antibiotic and germicidal qualities, and was often placed in sick rooms to help clear harmful bacteria. Honey also has anti-bacterial qualities, and soothes the inflamed mucous membrane.

16
THE URINARY SYSTEM

The urinary tract is a major elimination channel, filtering the bloodstream of its nitrogenous waste and excess salts.

The kidneys are two small bean-shaped organs situated about a third of the way up, and a few inches either side of, the spine. They produce the urine in which the waste is transported. When the kidneys are under-functioning, or when the amount of waste is too great for the kidneys to deal with efficiently, acid wastes start to build up inside the body.

The kidneys are called the seat of the emotions by the Chinese, and are particularly affected by anxiety and concern. If the kidneys are seen to be under-functioning in the iris, we can tell whether the cause is emotional and/or physical by investigating the diagonal reflex, the 'head' area of the iris being diagonally opposite the kidneys. In these circumstances, when the tissue in the head area has discolourations, the emotions will have been responsible, at least in part, for the weakened kidneys.

WEAK KIDNEYS AND/OR BLADDER

Where the kidneys and/or the bladder are weak, it is better to avoid all sulphuric foods (e.g. alcohol, hard cheeses, dried fruits containing sulphur dioxide, vinegars, battery-farmed eggs, etc.).

Contrary to popular opinion, it is not advisable to drink much fluid of any kind when the kidneys are weak or congested because this will only place them under additional strain – like trying to heal a broken leg by dancing on it. Drinking does not flush out the kidneys; it merely gives them more work to do. Even mineral water has to be filtered by the kidneys, to say nothing of the burden placed on them of having to filter out the pollutants in tap water. If one drinks anything it should be pure distilled water, freshly squeezed fruit and vegetable juices, or therapeutic herbal teas.

- Buchu is one herb that helps cleanse the kidneys.
- Avoid acid-forming foods.

Regular reflexology treatments will also help strengthen the kidneys and bladder, as will Chinese moxibustion.

INFLAMMATION

If the bladder is inflamed it can be flushed out by drinking fluid regularly and often, although with due consideration to the condition of the kidneys.

In cases of high acidity/inflammation avoid high acid-forming foods. Take slippery elm tablets (one/two with each meal), to absorb and eliminate excess acidity, and plenty of fresh grapes, eaten alone and as a meal, as these are high in alkalinity and very cleansing.

Barley water is an old remedy for cystitis (inflammation of the bladder, usually accompanied by an infection). Take 2–3 pints of the barley water, and drink it throughout the day.

Sodium phosphate is an acidity regulator, and helps in cases of inflammation in the kidney and bladder.

HEAVY CONGESTION IN THE KIDNEYS

When iris analysis shows the kidneys to be heavily congested it is advisable to follow the anti-acid diet strictly, and take several cups of an infusion of gravel root herb in place of coffee, throughout the day to help break up the crystal formations.

17
THE LYMPHATIC SYSTEM

Lymph is a fluid consisting of blood plasma (blood fluid without any blood cells) which has seeped through the capillaries in order to bathe and nourish the tissues. It then helps transport cellular wastes and harmful bacteria away from the tissues. The lymphatic system can therefore be likened to the waste disposal unit of the body, collecting dead cells, blood proteins and other toxic waste resulting from cellular activity throughout the body tissues, and transporting them, via the lymph nodes (where bacteria are killed), back into the bloodstream, from where the waste products are delivered to the various elimination channels.

All the body's cells rely upon the lymphatic system to drain off the toxic waste and excess fluids which, if left, would hinder the supply of oxygen to the tissues. In fact the lymphatic system is so crucial to your well-being that, if for some reason it stopped working, you would be dead from the blood poisoning within 24 hours.

So what makes the lymphatic system work? Well in many ways the lymphatic system is very similar to the vascular system (the arteries and veins), in that both are dependent on vessels that are stimulated by the muscular contraction of the tissues around them. Therefore, for the healthy functioning of the lymphatic system, exercise is again of the utmost importance. When a muscle flexes, the lymph vessel is squeezed and the lymph itself is moved towards the main lymph nodes, in the groin, armpits, neck, base of the lungs and in the abdomen. As the lymph passes through the lymph nodes, germs and toxic wastes can then be destroyed and neutralised.

A study by Dr Jack Shields in California suggests that deep diaphragmatic breathing is perhaps the most effective method of stimulating the flow of lymph through the body – as importantly as aerobic exercise. Dr Shields put cameras inside peoples' bodies to record how the lymph reacted to certain stimuli, and found that deep breathing created a sort of vacuum, sucking lymph through the lymphatic vessels and improving the rate of elimination of body wastes. In fact, when combined with exercise, deep breathing increased the cleansing process by 1,500 per cent.

Therefore, if the iris shows the lymph to be congested in one area or throughout the body, preventive action centres around diet, physical exercise and deep breathing.

CONGESTED LYMPH NODE(S)

If a part of the body is injured, germs begin to accumulate in and around the damaged tissues. Thankfully, the lymph collects the wastes and any bacteria and carries them to the lymph nodes, where they are trapped and prevented from spreading to other parts of the body. However, the more congested the lymphatic system becomes, the more susceptible the body is to infections, allergies and tissue abnormalities. It is therefore particularly important to ensure that any conditions seen in the iris as affecting the flow of lymph are dealt with before the immune system weakens and further health complications arise.

Where there are only one or two areas of congestion, there may be a physical obstruction causing it, in which case it is well worth a visit to a physical therapist to check it out. But if there is no physical obstruction, then the recommended health measures will be the same as for a complete rosary in the iris (see below).

If deep congestion appears in the breast region, it is advisable to consult your physician for further examination, and also adhere strictly to the preventive measures outlined for a complete rosary.

LYMPHATIC ROSARY

Where congestion is seen in the form of a lymphatic rosary, it indicates that the patient has a weakened immune system. As a result, cellular waste is able to accumulate inside the body. This requires preventive measures as it can precipitate pathological disease. The darker the rosary, the more chronic and deep-seated is the congestion.

Remedial measures
In all instances where the flow of lymph is sluggish, the following measures are advisable.

Avoid mucus-forming foods Red meats, dairy foods (especially hard cheeses), refined white sugar products and wheat products are all highly mucus-forming and create further congestion in the body. It is therefore prudent to avoid these foods or, at the very least, keep them to a minimum.

Avoid refined sugar products Six teaspoons of refined white sugar deplete the body of 25 per cent of its white blood cells, therefore making us more susceptible to infection.

Eat plenty of fresh fruits and vegetables It is the water-rich foods – the fresh fruits, vegetables and sprouted beans – that cleanse the blood and lymph. We are made up of the same elements as the earth, and in very similar proportions. Just as the earth is approximately 70 per cent water, so are we, and to maintain that balance our diet should therefore contain approximately 70 per cent water. And not just any water, but pure water, none being so pure as that found in the water-rich foods.

The importance of water-rich foods was highlighted in the findings of Dr Alexander Bryce, who states in *The Laws of Life and Health* that:

When too little fluid is supplied, the blood maintains a higher specific gravity and the poisonous waste products of tissue or cell change are only cast off very imperfectly. The body is, therefore, poisoned by its own excretions, and it is not too much to say that the chief reason of this is because a sufficient amount of fluid has not been supplied to carry off in solution the waste matter the cells manufacture.

Stimulating the flow of lymph

Deep diaphragmatic breathing As we noted previously, deep breathing and general exercise are the most efficient ways to stimulate the lymphatic system; these are described in detail in Chapter 15, which deals with the respiratory system.

What is important to realise is that if you perform the exercises regularly you will slowly build up your lung capacity and help cleanse the lymphatic system. In time you will instinctively breathe more and more deeply.

Remedial massage Regular remedial massage is also an excellent way of stimulating both lymphatic and blood circulation. The manipulation of the soft tissues physically encourages the flow of lymph through the vessels towards the lymph nodes.

Skin brushing Skin brushing with a hard-bristled brush will have a similar effect to that of massage, although unlike massage, it will not relax the tissues or sooth away tensions. However skin brushing is effective in stimulating the flow of lymph, and is something that we can all do quickly and easily as it takes no more than a few moments of your time (see pages 263–4).

Footbaths and saunas Hot and cold footbaths are again recommended to stimulate blood and lymph circulation. If possible, regular saunas will also improve the circulation and encourage elimination of toxins through the skin.

A NOTE OF CAUTION

Stimulating the lymphatic system can cause reactions in other elimination channels, especially the bowels and skin, as the body may not be able to cope with the rapid elimination of accumulated toxins. It is similar to too much rubbish being poured down a drain; only so much can pass at one time without the drain becoming blocked. Consequently, constipation and minor skin complaints may sometimes occur if too much waste is eliminated into the intestines or skin. Therefore whenever cleansing the lymphatic system, it is always advisable to take a herbal bowel tonic in conjunction with the aforementioned treatments, in order to ensure regular movement of the bowels.

18
THE MUSCULAR–SKELETAL SYSTEM

Structure affects function.

F.M. Alexander

The muscular–skeletal system is perhaps the most important system in the body, because every organ is dependent in some way or another on muscular contraction. Without muscles we would not be able to walk, talk, see or even breathe. In short, without muscles we could not live.

MUSCLES AND ORGANS

If you were to watch an abdominal operation you would see that all of the internal organs are moving rhythmically inside the abdomen, each to a particular rhythm created by the tissue around it. But when an organ malfunctions the rhythm changes, becoming faster if the organ is inflamed and slower if the organ is degenerating. And the reverse is also true. If the tissue around the organ disturbs the rhythm, the functioning of the organ will change accordingly. A good example is that of a kidney infection, which causes the muscles in the back to go into spasm, creating pain. Yet, conversely, if the kidney is functioning well but the same muscles in the mid to lower back go into spasm, the functioning of the kidney will be affected.

Many people sit all day in sedentary occupations, and this allows the diaphragm to become lazy. As a result, the

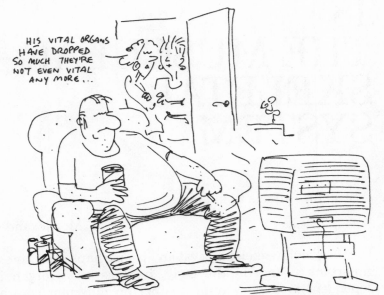

SITTING DOWN ALL DAY WITHOUT EXERCISE CAUSES THE VITAL ORGANS WITHIN THE ABDOMINAL CAVITY TO DROP OUT OF THEIR ORIGINAL POSITIONS...

lungs are under-utilised and stale air accumulates in them. Sitting down all day without any exercise also causes the abdominal wall to sag and the vital organs within the abdominal cavity to drop out of their original positions (a condition called visceroptosis). The organs therefore lose their natural rhythm, and consequently their proper functions are adversely affected.

MUSCLES AND JOINTS

The muscles, tendons and ligaments hold the joints and bones in the body together. If a muscle is damaged, the related joint will be pulled out of place and this may obstruct the blood and/or nerve supply to other parts of the body.

For instance, the central nervous system stems from the spinal cord, which is protected by the vertebrae (the bones in the spine). If muscles on one side of the back are damaged, vertebrae will become displaced due to the fact that the damaged muscles on one side of the spine have a weaker pull than the muscles on the other side. The nerve root which stems from between the vertebrae will also be restricted; as all tissue is only as healthy as the blood that is supplied to it and the nerve that enervates it, it follows that a restricted nerve will adversely affect the tissue it enervates.

Healthy blood and nerve supply require free unrestricted blood vessels and nerve pathways, which can only be ensured by correct posture, which in turn can only be achieved through balanced muscles. Postural distortions create distortions of blood flow and nerve supply, tissues thereby become weak and undernourished, and dis-ease sets in.

Therefore if the soft tissues are balanced, the joints will be in their correct positions, the nerve and blood supply will be unrestricted, and all the body tissues will be kept healthy.

INFLAMMATION

Any physical injury or trauma will cause inflammation. If you fall over, bang your arm, or receive a kick during a football game, there will be inflammation, including swelling, around the physical injury. The swelling is part of the body's own healing process; a large proportion of any swelling consists of blood fluids and lymph, which bathe and nourish the damaged tissues before eliminating the cellular waste.

In all cases of physical injury it is advisable to see a physical therapist or other health practitioner because, even when the symptoms go, there may be residual effects which will lead to other problems if left neglected. For instance, a minor muscular strain in the lower back, if untreated, may merely cause pain now and again – nothing much to worry about you might think. But slowly the lumbar vertebrae could be pulled out of their correct position, and what was a small muscular injury, over the years, could become a chronic joint disorder, with wear on the intra-vertebral discs.

However there are simple measures that you can take which help the body's healing processes after an injury, and often circumvent the need for treatment. The easy way to remember what to do in all cases of muscular injury is to keep the word RICE in your mind.

- **R** = rest. Rest the injured limb or area. Take all pressure and strain off the area to allow the body's healing process to work as efficiently as possible. Further strain leads to further pain, and worsens the original damage.
- **I** = ice. Ice packs (a packet of frozen peas will do the job nicely) should be placed on the injured area for 10–15 minutes when it is angry and inflamed, and repeated every 4–5 hours. If there is no redness, you can substitute the ice packs with hot and cold packs (hot-water bottle and an ice pack) – hot for three minutes followed by cold for one minute, repeated two or three times. This will increase blood and lymph flow to the area; increase the number of white blood cells and metabolism in the area; and help prevent adhesions forming (fibres sticking together), all thereby stimulating the healing process.
- **C** = compression. Wrap the area in a bandage to prevent further swelling. The bandage should not be so tight as to cause pain; remember, the swelling is the body's natural reaction and part of the healing process, directing blood fluids and lymph to the injured area to bathe and nourish it. But our sedentary lifestyle encourages the body to over-compensate, and the larger the swelling, the longer it will take for the area to get back to its original state.
- **E** = elevation. Keep the limb or area elevated to allow easy flow of blood and lymph away from the area. In many cases poor circulation is the cause of the formation of adhesions; the lymph becomes sticky and then

hardens, joining muscular fibres together. Once adhesions are formed they have to be broken down, and this can take months.

In acute cases of physical trauma, and where there is deep bruising and pain, give arnica tablets (two tablets six times for one day and then three times a day, not with food or coffee/tea) and apply arnica ointment to the area. In cases of nerve damage take hypericum tablets (as for arnica).

Inflammation caused by excess acidity

A build up of acid in the tissues may not be the result of an injury; it may be caused by having a high proportion of acid-forming foods in the diet, as these also create joint and muscle inflammation. When this happens, however, the inflammation is usually spread over the body rather than in one location.

If this is the case, it is advisable to avoid high acid-forming foods (see page 264) and instead eat more cleansing and alkaline foods such as fresh fruit (except citrus fruit, strawberries and rhubarb), especially fresh grapes and melons, and vegetables (except cooked tomatoes and cooked spinach).

It is also advisable to take slippery elm tablets (one with each meal, to help eliminate the acidity) and sodium phosphate.

LOOSE TISSUE

Loose tissue indicates weakness in the connective tissue in the affected part of the body and it is in such areas that one tends to develop muscular/skeletal problems. For example, if there is loose connective tissue in the lower back, that will be the site of injury if posture and exercise are neglected and it is not uncommon for people to have loose tissue on the right side of the neck and shoulders, due to the fact that their necks are continuously bent to the left, holding the phone, during hours of work at the office. Therefore to remedy the situation you can simply hold the phone at times on the right side of your neck, or alternatively at intervals during the day stretch the neck to the right.

Exercise

Whether or not there is loose tissue in a section of the spine or elsewhere in the body, it is always advisable to do regular exercise; however, this is of even greater importance where loose tissue is in evidence. So you must do some form of daily exercise. Find something that you enjoy doing, which will make the heart beat a little faster and produce perspiration. Brisk walking and swimming for 20 minutes are excellent forms of exercise for the body.

Chapter 27 on posture and exercise in Part III of the book contains a general exercise programme designed to improve blood circulation and encourage mobility and flexibility, and so tone up the muscles.

A word of warning With any exercise programme, take care not to overdo it. Never go beyond the point of pain, and remember to build up slowly. If you have a history of heart-related disorders consult your doctor before beginning any exercise programme.

19
THE DIGESTIVE SYSTEM

Good nutrition is the first step to good health. However it is not just what we eat that is important. You can eat the best food in the world and still digest it or eliminate it imperfectly. So nutrition is not just about food, nor just about minerals, vitamins and other nutrients. It is about the ability of the body to absorb and utilise those nutrients and then eliminate the waste – in other words, it is about the whole digestive process.

DIGESTION

Digestion begins in the mouth and ends at the rectum. The stomach and intestines are essentially a long tube inside the body, within which the foods we eat are broken down into nutrients to be absorbed and assimilated into the bloodstream, and then fed to the tissues throughout the body. The whole digestive process thus depends not just on the food we eat but also when we eat it, how we eat it and, of course, on the condition of the digestive organs and their ability to break down the food and to absorb the nutrients.

For instance, the metabolism and digestion generally slow down in the evening; therefore food eaten in the evening will not be as efficiently digested as food eaten in the morning. Similarly, eating between meals retards digestion. The stomach does not function like a conveyor belt. It is more like a mixing bowl, in which foods are broken down and prepared for absorption through the small intestines. A normal meal may take between 2–6 hours to pass through the stomach, but if you eat a snack between meals the stomach stops mixing and starts all over again. So food that ordinarily would pass through the stomach in a few hours, stays in the stomach for up to 15 hours, during which time it putrefies and ferments, causing wind; it then passes into the small intestines improperly broken down, and cannot be efficiently absorbed.

Exercise is also very important in maintaining the peristaltic muscular movement of the colon wall – sluggish abdominal muscles lead to a sluggish colon. So make sure you do some form of regular exercise, even if it is only a few miles of brisk walking every day.

Emotions affect the digestive organs. Digestive organs under-function when you are under emotional strain. Who hasn't felt their stomach and intestines knotting up when suffering emotional turmoil? In these circumstances you can eat like a horse, but you still won't put on any weight. And why? Because the food hasn't been properly digested. Toxins can then accumulate within the body, so you may end up with skin complaints, migraines, abdominal pain, constipation and a host of other symptoms.

Healthy digestion of course depends upon the actual state of your stomach and intestines and digestive organs. For example, if you have hyper-acidity or even stomach ulcers you will not be able to digest oranges or peanuts very well; these and other acid-forming foods will therefore often cause pain. Similarly, if you have a weak gall bladder you will not be able to digest fatty foods well. If your pancreas is congested you will not be able to convert carbohydrates and high sugar foods into energy efficiently. And so the list goes on.

Efficient and healthy digestion therefore depends upon:

- The food we eat.
- How and when we eat it.
- The state of the digestive system.

Iris analysis reveals the state of the digestive system, and from there you can find out those foods that are best for you and those foods you would do better to avoid.

BOWEL TOXAEMIA

A toxic state in the digestive tract is a common condition, prohibiting efficient digestion and often leading to lethargy as a result of the inability to absorb nutrients fully. It may be caused by a poor diet, by excessive use of medications (particularly antibiotics), many of which kill off the protective flora in the intestines, and by negative emotions, which hinder the digestive process. It is important to remember that the liver will also be under-functioning, due to the fact that it is the liver's job to filter out the accumulated toxins from the bloodstream.

In such a case a herbal cleansing programme is advisable. It is best carried out for a period of three months, and repeated on a yearly basis if necessary. This will help to cleanse the entire digestive tract and break down any hardened faecal matter that may have accumulated in the colon, as well as helping to heal, tone and strengthen the lower intestinal tract.

Bowel cleansing formula 1

This has a gentle cleansing action and a soothing laxative effect, designed to deal with cases where the toxaemia is accompanied by constipation.

It consists of a combination of mandrake root, ginger, liquorice root, calamus root, cayenne, cascara sagrada bark, wild yam root and calendula. One ounce of each powdered herb is mixed together with hard-set honey until it forms a doughy consistency. Two pieces of this dough, the size of a pea, may then be taken with food three times a day.

This dosage is designed to restore normal bowel motions. However the dosage should be monitored according to changes in the bowel movements, e.g. if the stools are too loose then reduce the dosage, and in chronic cases of constipation increase the dosage by up to 10 times, until stools pass easily and are a well-formed sausage shape.

In addition, one level teaspoon of psyllium husk should be mixed in a large tumbler of fruit juice and/or water, and drunk immediately prior to each meal. Psyllium expands in fluid and turns into a soft jelly in the stomach and intestines, where it acts like a gentle broom, sweeping out old faecal matter from the intestinal tract. (This is also very useful in cases of haemorrhoids.)

Cleansing formula 2
This formula has a slightly stronger herbal combination, and may be used when the toxaemia is not accompanied by chronic constipation, or when the constipation subsides. It consists of a combination of centaury (a liver cleanser), cactus grand, calendula and dandelion, and is designed to stimulate the liver, cleanse the blood and soothe inflammation in, and help clear accumulated waste from, the intestinal tract.

HYPER-ACIDITY

Excess acid in the alimentary tract is caused by too many acid forming foods and/or negative emotions. Therefore changing the diet and sorting out any emotional disturbances are a prerequisite to overcoming this condition.

One patient of mine had extremely bright white discolouring in the stomach and intestinal zones of the iris, indicating terribly high levels of acidity. Sure enough, questioning revealed that he suffered from stomach ulcers and colitis (an inflamed colon). As part of his treatment he avoided all acid-forming foods, and for the first time in over five years he was able to come off his steroids. However he could not overcome the antagonism he felt towards his wife, and every time he had a confrontation with her his colitis flared up.

Herbs
Slippery elm is the inner lining of the bark of an elm tree,

and absorbs excess acidity and soothes inflammations. In all cases of excess acidity or inflammation one should avoid high acid-forming foods and take slippery elm tablets, one with each meal, to absorb and eliminate acid. In severe cases one glass of raw cabbage juice taken daily will also help, even to the extent of healing ulcers.

Herb teas made from chamomile (relaxant) and comfrey (soothes inflammation) can be taken in place of tea/coffee, both of which are high acid forming drinks. A herbal infusion of comfrey (anti-inflammatory), meadow sweet (blood cleanser), elderflower (blood cleanser) and buchu (kidney cleanser) is a pleasant tasting tea and always help in the elimination of accumulated acidity from the alimentary tract (see page 186 for how to make herbal infusions).

Fruit and vegetables

Raw fruits, and raw vegetables and salads are best put through a blender or chewed thoroughly, otherwise the hard cellulose from the plant cell walls may irritate the stomach and intestines. Fruits and vegetables should not be eaten at the same meal, as the acids are incompatible and can cause irritation.

HYPO-ACIDITY

The much rarer condition of insufficient acid in the stomach and intestines is usually caused by enzyme deficiency. Once signs of hypo-acidity appear in the iris it is therefore time to check your diet and emotions.

A mono-diet (i.e. eating only one food at a meal) for a week gives the stomach a much needed rest and takes the strain off the stomach acid secretions. Simple foods are most favourable, with little or no spices, and plenty of goat's milk yoghurt or acidophilis capsules are recommended to restore the protective flora in the intestines.

If there are any adverse symptoms, consult a health practitioner for a full examination.

SPASTIC COLON

A spastic colon (in which the wall of the large intestine loses its tone and becomes slack and mis-shapen) is often caused by a poor diet with inadequate roughage. However changing the diet to include more fibrous wholesome foods should be gradual, particularly if there are faecal impactions in the diverticula (pockets) of the colon wall.

Psyllium husk, the soft soluble fibre mentioned earlier, helps restore tone to the colon wall, while plenty of barley, rice, oats and lightly steamed vegetables provide soft bulk which slowly tones and cleanses the intestinal walls and thereby helps restore the normal peristaltic motion of the colon.

TIGHT COLON

Tension in the colon wall narrows the diameter of the large intestine through which the faeces move, and often creates constipation. Chronic constipation in turn leads to chronic toxaemia and chronic degenerative diseases.

The bowels should ideally move once for each meal; certainly anything less than one movement a day falls within the definition of constipation. But even if the bowels are moving regularly there may still be constipation if, for instance, one is straining to pass a stool.

A tight colon may be caused by a diet largely consisting of refined food products. However there is often an emotional cause, so any unresolved emotional conflicts must usually be dealt with before any real progress can be made. Herbal tranquillisers (see pages 179–80) and Bach flower remedies are often successful in helping in the treatment of emotional problems.

Chamomile tea is a widely used relaxant, while preparations containing magnesium phosphate will also help relax the tightness of the tissues in the colon wall.

IMPACTIONS

Old faecal matter stuck to the inner wall of the intestines is usually due to sluggish movement in the bowels, as a result of which too much fluid is re-absorbed through the colon wall. The faeces then become sticky and hard and cling to the colon wall, causing putrefaction and fermentation. This will also create reflex effects in other parts of the body, depending upon the location of the impaction (see Chapter 6 on reflexes in the eyes).

Whenever impactions are detected in the iris a herbal bowel cleanse is advisable to deal with them. An appropriate treatment is the bowel formula 1 or 2 cleanse (see pages 167-8), depending upon whether impaction is accompanied by constipation or not.

THE MAIN DIGESTIVE ORGANS

The three major organs to be considered in the digestive process are the liver, gall bladder and pancreas.

The liver

The liver is the largest gland in the body, with over 500 known functions. It is therefore not surprising that when the liver is under-functioning the body will suffer in a multitude of ways, primarily from the accumulation of toxicity within the tissues, particularly in the stomach and intestines. This is because one of the liver's primary tasks is to filter toxins.

In all cases of toxicity and where the liver is congested, one should therefore take the herb centaury. This can be taken in tablet form, as directed on page 259, or made into a tea and drunk cold first thing in the morning. The reason for taking the tea cold is that the herb is terribly bitter and most people find it undrinkable when hot; drunk cold, however, much of the bitterness cannot be tasted.

Gall bladder

The gall bladder stores bile, which is involved in the digestion of fats. High consumption of saturated fats puts a strain on the gall bladder and causes a build up of cholesterol within the body. Therefore a diet low in saturated fats (e.g. low in all meats, hard cheeses, butter and other dairy produce) is essential where the iris shows the gall bladder to be under-functioning or congested.

Lecithin is a food substance obtained from soy beans and sunflower seeds. It is a well-known emulsifier and as such can help to break down fats. One tablespoon of lecithin granules may therefore be taken with each meal, on its own or sprinkled on cereal, soups or gravy, or mixed with a glass of fruit juice and drunk before the meal.

Plenty of garlic and onions, freshly squeezed fruit and vegetable juices, freshly chopped salads, and extra virgin cold-pressed olive oil all have a beneficial effect on the digestion of fats, while oats eaten regularly have been shown to reduce cholesterol levels. All these steps will help take some stress off the gall bladder.

Pancreas

The pancreas has two particularly important functions in the digestive process:

- The secretion of pancreatic juices to help break down proteins.
- The secretion of insulin to control the sugar level in the blood.

High protein foods and high sugar foods put a strain on the pancreas, and can cause a build-up of toxins and the gradual weakening of the organ. So if the iris indicates that the pancreas is congested or weak, it is sensible to avoid all high-protein foods, including all meats and hard cheeses, and essential to avoid all sweet foods, especially those containing refined sugar.

Instead, a cleansing diet high in fresh vegetables and fruits is recommended, including plenty of Jerusalem artichokes, adzuki beans, potimarrons (similar to pumpkin), garlic and onions, all of which have been shown to have a beneficial effect on the pancreas and the blood-sugar levels.

Where diabetes has been clinically diagnosed and insulin injections are prescribed, it is recommended that you consult your health practitioner before changing your diet in any way.

20
THE ENDOCRINE SYSTEM

The endocrine system consists of the glands within the body which secrete substances (mainly hormones) required for certain bodily functions. The glands produce precise and often minute amounts of substances at specific times; for instance, in the evening most of nature slows down and hormones are secreted in the body to slow down our metabolic rate. When we turn night into day by going out at all hours the hormonal balance becomes distorted and slowly an imbalance occurs. Erratic lifestyles are thus harmful to the endocrine system; the body has its own clock and we should stick to it whenever possible.

The endocrine system looms particularly large in women's consciousness today, as many middle-aged women are increasingly faced with the awkward decision of whether or not to take hormone replacement therapy (HRT) to cope with adverse menopausal symptoms. Indeed, many women are now being advised to take HRT, even though they are not suffering from any symptoms, simply as a 'preventive' measure to help avoid the development of osteoporosis (brittle bones) in later years.

Bearing in mind that there have been no long-term studies on the possible side effects of HRT, and that most studies that have been carried out on the subject conflict in their findings, this advice seems at the very least questionable. The main discrepancies between the studies relates to the extent of the possible damage to health such drugs might induce: some studies have found that HRT might increase the risk of strokes; others find it might increase the risk of various forms of cancer (some by up to ten times), and the risk does not diminish if the patient stops taking the drug. In all, it would appear that taking HRT to avoid brittle bones is like cutting your head off to get rid of a headache.

However, in this chapter we are primarily concerned with the master gland (the pituitary gland), the adrenal gland and the thyroid gland.

THE PITUITARY GLAND

The pituitary gland, very simply, controls all the endocrine glands in the body.

The pituitary is often affected by impaction/toxicity in the transverse colon, in which case the colon needs to be cleansed (see page 167). If this is the case, the first thing to do is regulate the diet and make sure that all meats are avoided, as they are often heavily contaminated with hormones. Eat regularly, and try not to turn night into day and day into night.

If the iris indicates a disturbance with the gland itself, it is worth visiting your local practitioner as natural preventive treatments are far safer and preferable to the use of drugs.

THE THYROID GLAND

The thyroid gland controls the body's metabolism (the conversion of food into energy), and is particularly susceptible to weak tissue, congestion, hyperactivity, etc. To minimise these risks one should eat regular meals, and the evening meal should be light rather than heavy. Kelp tablets are good for strengthening the thyroid gland, as they are high in iodine – an essential nutrient for the thyroid.

Where the iris appears to show deep congestion, and there are adverse symptoms of general tiredness, a herbal mixture consisting of powdered parsley leaves, kelp, Irish moss, Iceland moss, nettles, bladderwrack and bugleweed, mixed in equal quantities, usually helps.

THE ADRENAL GLANDS

Known as fight or flight glands, the adrenals are well known as being essential for dealing with stress. Perhaps less well known is their role in combating inflammatory illnesses; the cortex, the centre, of the adrenals produces cortisone, the body's anti-inflammatory chemical, which helps cope with all injuries.

The adrenals are therefore affected by emotional tension, frustration and suppressed rage. Where a disturbance of the adrenals is seen in the iris, it is time to rest; to step away from confrontations and emotional stresses; to ensure a balanced nutritious diet; and perhaps to take a herbal tonic.

21
THE NERVOUS SYSTEM

The nervous system is a finely woven and extremely intricate system of nerve pathways through which the brain sends and receives messages throughout the body. It is an electrical powerhouse that stimulates the function of every organ in the body without which no muscle would be able to contract, the stomach wouldn't know when it needed to be filled, and the lungs wouldn't be able to breathe. In sum, each of the body systems would 'shut down' if the nervous system stopped functioning.

It is commonly accepted that most diseases in the so-called civilised world are caused, at least in part, by stress. A strained nervous system is often the beginning of other physical and psychological disorders – stomach ulcers, colitis, irritable bowels, skin complaints, migraines, high blood pressure, muscular tension, arthritis, eye strain. Likewise, stress may lead to hypertension, insomnia, anxiety and depression. However, all ailments, save those caused by physical trauma or injury, will have been caused, at least in part, by some form of emotional stress; for emotional stress always leads to physical stress, and in the first instance affects the weakest and most vulnerable parts of the body.

The first signs of nervous strain will appear in the iris. You will thus be given an advance warning of impending problems, and will be able to take action accordingly.

DIETARY FACTORS

Most of us put unnecessary strain on our nervous systems through improper diet. For example, vitamin B is one of the most vital of nutrients as far as the nervous system is concerned, yet common foods and drinks such as coffee, tea, refined flour products, chocolate, colas, and all products containing white sugar, deplete the body of vitamin B complex.

Sucrose quickly raises the blood-sugar level, giving an initial boost of energy, but this is quickly followed by irritability and mood fluctuations as the blood-sugar level rapidly drops to a lower level to where it had been initially.

Eating a heavy meal late in the evening also leads to nervous strain. The brain has to work all night, sending and receiving messages to and from the stomach and intestines, in order to coordinate the digestion of the food. Consequently one awakes in the morning feeling tired instead of refreshed.

During periods of stress it is therefore important to give your diet special attention, and to try to avoid as much as possible those foods and dietary considerations which put added strain on the nervous system. Vitamin B complex tablets will help, but should not be relied upon as most vitamin tablets are made up synthetically and are not properly absorbed by the body. As I mentioned earlier, it is much better to obtain nutrients from wholesome food than man-made potions or tablets.

TENSION RINGS

When tension rings are seen in the iris it indicates accumulated emotional stress resulting in physical tension throughout the connective tissue in the body. However the cause of this is not really stress as such, but our reactions to certain stresses. For instance, two people may be travelling to work on the same train, which is held up, causing both men to be late. One man gets agitated, starts pulling his hair out and raising his blood pressure by ten points. In contrast the other man says to himself 'I can't make the train go any faster, and getting uptight about it won't remedy the situation', he remains calm, using the time more constructively by taking a mental check of the tasks ahead of him.

To prevent strain on the nervous system we must free ourselves of internal emotional conflict. Of course, you may say, this is more easily said than done; but the fact remains that, as far as our mind and thoughts are concerned, we are in control. No one can make us feel depressed, rejected or upset; only we decide how we react to what others say or do around us. Therefore our attitudes may need to be looked at and, if necessary, changed if they are to be conducive to our happiness.

For instance, if you get bored and depressed every time you go to work, ask yourself why. Then, when you have found the answer, take some action to remedy it. The sources of all problems must be removed, before they have time to fester and destroy you. Chapter 28 lists examples and techniques for changing your perspectives and attitudes, so that you can adopt a more positive outlook – one that may be more conducive, not just to controlling the effects of stress but also, simply, to being happy.

However there are several other ways this condition may be helped and reversed.

Herbal remedies

Natural herbs such as valerian root, chamomile, cramp bark and lady's slipper are well-known traditional herbal relaxants.

- Valerian root has a mild soothing effect on the nervous system, and aids mental relaxation.
- Lady's slipper is a much stronger herb, particularly helpful when taken before bed in order to overcome even the most stubborn cases of insomnia.
- Cramp bark, on the other hand, helps relieve physical tension and release spasms within the body.
- Chamomile is a gentle calmative to soothe the nerves; it is easily available and quite pleasant taken as a tea.

All four herbs will help to calm the system down in times of intense stress, and none of them is known to have any unpleasant side effects. But remember that anything taken in excess will be harmful, so stick to recommended doses.

Relaxation and visualisation techniques

Deep breathing techniques, sitting or lying down in a comfortable position and listening to a relaxation tape of soft music will help to calm down the system.

Try giving yourself a five-minute 'mind holiday' every day. Simply visualise yourself relaxing on a beach, beside a lake, or wherever takes your fancy. These five minutes away from the stresses and strains of your daily life, allowing yourself to unwind, albeit for a short time, will give tremendous benefits.

Massage

There is nothing like a good massage to soothe away all the stresses and strains of the day. A massage can significantly bring down high blood pressure, by over 20 points. Furthermore, the soothing strokes relax and calm the nervous system, whilst physically easing the accumulated physical tension. Knotted-up confused emotions create knotted-up connective tissues and muscles in the body; conversely, relaxing the muscles will likewise relax the mind.

Ultimately, though, you must tackle the cause of the stress or the reasons why you have allowed the tension to accumulate.

SMALL PUPILS

A tight small pupil indicates that the person is going through a stressful time, and the herbal tranquillisers and relaxants mentioned above will greatly help in such circumstances and prevent any build up of anxiety or stress within the body.

However, as a person with a small pupil is under stress, it is advisable to ensure that he or she is well nourished, eating a balanced wholefood diet and drinking freshly squeezed fruit and vegetable juices for additional easily absorbed nutrients. This is far preferable to synthetic vitamin and mineral tablets. It is also important to avoid taking stimulants such as tea, coffee and alcohol, and refined white sugar products, as these will deplete the body of vitamin B and other nutrients necessary to sustain the nervous system.

Fluid extract of valerian root will help relax the mind without causing drowsiness, and products containing magnesium phosphate helps relieve the physical tension and tightness in the body's tissues.

DILATED PUPILS

A large pupil indicates nervous exhaustion, a depletion of nervous energy. The person will probably have been through a period of stress and will have used up all their reserves of nervous energy. Remedial measures will include the following:

Nutrition

First and foremost, it is important to ensure a simple yet wholesome nutritious diet so that the nervous system is adequately nourished. Plenty of fresh fruit and vegetables, all of which are easily digested, together with sprouted seeds, and fresh vegetable and fruit juices, the nutrients of which are absorbed within 10–15 minutes, should be the mainstay. Blackstrap molasses, extracted from sugar cane, is extremely rich in iron and essential minerals; one teaspoon stirred in hot water with a slice of lemon is an excellent nutritious tonic.

At times of depleted energy it is tempting to resort to tea with sugar, chocolates and other sweets. Don't! These will quickly raise the blood-sugar level, giving an initial feeling of energy, but this will equally quickly fade away and leave you worse off than when you started. This is due to the fact that, in order for the body to convert refined sugars into energy, it needs the minerals and elements that would accompany the sugar in nature. As all such nutrients have been excluded in the refining process, the body has to resort to taking these elements from its own tissues. Similarly, stimulants such as coffee, tea and alcohol quickly wear off, leaving you exhausted in the long run.

Herbs

Herbal fluid extracts of black cohosh, blue cohosh, ginger and skullcap act as a superb tonic in times of nervous exhaustion, stimulating the nervous system.

Hot and cold footbaths

Alternating hot and cold footbaths serve to stimulate the blood and lymphatic circulation, not just in the feet but throughout the whole body. They thus have a superb tonic effect, strengthening the entire body.

This is an old yet wonderful form of hydrotherapy, easily carried out in your own home, and taking little more than 10 minutes (see page 261).

Moxibustion

The burning of the Chinese herb called moxa over specified acupuncture points gives energy to the body organs and systems. This is an absolutely fabulous tonic, and works through stimulating the various meridians or flows of energy in the body – a simple and safe method of energising the body.

Rest and rejuvenation

What is really needed to restore the body's strength and nervous energy is simply physical rest and mental relaxation – a time to slow down, take a break from the pressures that have been building up and become carefree (as opposed to careless), even if only for a while.

It is written that 'man does not live by bread alone'; we do not just get energy from the food we eat, but also from our emotions. Haven't you noticed that when you are enthusiastic about someone or something, when you are in love or when you receive wonderful news, you feel energised and unstoppable? You can recreate this feeling any time you want by recalling in your mind a time when you felt really good and on top of the world, perhaps repeating the actions you would normally do in those situations. I like to clench my fists and shout, 'Yes', as if I had just scored the winning goal in the World Cup final. Whatever action you do when you feel energised, you can repeat whenever you feel below par, and immediately you will feel energised.

THE AUTONOMIC NERVE WREATH

The ANW reveals how the emotional and physical stresses have affected the condition of the nervous system. Nervous stress, like physical stress can be tolerated, and is even beneficial up to a point; but beyond that point it will start to interfere with the strength of the nervous system, causing irritation, and in some cases degeneration.

As with all conditions affecting the nervous system, dietary measures need to be considered and emotional conflicts removed. However the ANW is intimately connected to the stomach and intestines and it is therefore also important to ensure that the digestive system is functioning well.

An inflamed nerve wreath in the head area of an iris indicates a mind full of concern and worry, and these need to be let go of. Worries, feelings of guilt, resentments, are just a few of the things that play on the mind and end up irritating the nervous system. Instead of concentrating on problems, it is better to concentrate on solutions, and if no solution comes to mind, simply let go and pray about it.

22
THE CARDIO-VASCULAR SYSTEM

The life of the body is in the blood.

Leviticus 17, 11

The cardio-vascular system carries the lifestream of the body, transporting vital nutrients all over the body, eliminating cellular waste and defending the tissues from invading bacteria.

The heart is only a small pear-shaped hollow muscle and yet it is the strongest and most important muscle in the body (save for the uterus in women, which only has to work really hard when a woman gives birth). The heart works at least twice as hard as the leg muscles of an Olympic 100-metre sprinter, which would very quickly turn to jelly under similar strain. In an average adult the heart has to pump blood through 60,000 miles of vessels every day. Freshly oxygenated blood is being continuously pumped through the arteries all over the body, carrying nutrients to nourish and cleanse the body tissues, and removing cellular waste.

The red cells in the blood carry oxygen from the lungs to the tissues of the body and then transport waste carbon dioxide from the tissues back to the lungs. The white blood cells (leucocytes) defend the body by fighting off invading bacteria and viruses. These, and the platelets responsible for blood clotting, all have to be transported around the body in the cardio-vascular system.

Circulation is thus vital to energy and general health; as

circulation fails, energy fails. As Dr Thomas Cureton, a former head of the physical fitness laboratory at the University of Illinois, has put it:

> Good circulation is the key to maximum health and energy ... the fight is mainly to keep the capillaries open ... otherwise a person grows old prematurely. He becomes introverted, with tendencies to anxiety, over-sensitiveness, and mental fatigue.

To keep the body healthy we must therefore keep the bloodstream healthy and active because no germ can survive in a pure bloodstream. And the iris provides a clear picture of what is going on in the circulatory system.

SCURF RIM

A scurf rim in the iris indicates poor arterial blood circulation; as a result, people with this problem often experience cold hands and feet. It is also associated with minor skin complaints (e.g. dermatitis, eczema, psoriasis, acne, etc.), due to the lack of nutrients reaching the skin and inefficient elimination of waste from and through the skin.

Where a scurf rim is visible in the iris it is advisable, whether or not any of the above symptoms have been experienced, to:

- Improve blood circulation.
- Improve elimination through the skin.
- Ensure that all other elimination channels (i.e. bowels, kidneys, lungs and lymph) are functioning well; when one elimination channel is blocked, the others will try to compensate and eventually the excess burden will cause them to suffer as well.

Improve blood circulation

Blood circulation can be improved in several ways, among which are the following:

Exercise Poor blood circulation is often caused by lack of exercise. The heart is simply a hollow muscular organ and, like other muscle tissue in the body, if it is not exercised it will start to weaken and then be unable to pump the blood through the tissues as well as it should. Furthermore, the contraction of muscles all over the body, but particularly in the legs, is responsible for squeezing the blood up through the veins and back to the heart – the flow of blood through the veins in the legs has to fight against gravity, so exercise is consequently crucial to maintaining good blood circulation.

Whether it be a brisk 20-minute walk in the park, a cycle ride in the country, or swimming 10 lengths of an Olympic-sized swimming pool, daily exercise is essential; without it the blood circulation will quickly suffer.

Hot and cold footbaths These are a wonderful tonic and will stimulate blood and lymphatic circulation, not just to the feet but all over the body (see page 261).

Herbal remedies Herbal remedies are not a cure-all to stimulate blood circulation, and are certainly no substitute for regular physical exercise. However there are two herbs in particular, cactus grand and liquorice root, that are renowned for their beneficial effect on blood circulation. Both may be taken as a tea; as with all herbal tea infusions, use one teaspoon per cup, and infuse for five minutes. It is always advisable to start with weaker rather than stronger tea, not just so that you can get used to the taste, but also because strong herbal tea can have a strong effect and produce a cleansing reaction. Weaker tea has a gentler effect; as the body starts to cleanse itself you can then start to make the tea stronger. (For the making of herbal remedies see page 257).

Avoid smoking Smoking cigarettes, apart from its effect on the other body systems, is one of the most destructive habits as far as the cardio-vascular system is concerned. Cigarette smoking has the effect of constricting the capillaries and thereby severely hindering free blood circulation throughout the body.

ARCUS SENILIS

The arcus senilis, the whitish ring around the arterial zone of the iris, indicates hardening of the arteries, and is a common condition, particularly in elderly people. Of perhaps more concern is the fact that it is becoming increasingly common in younger and middle-aged people.

Hardening of the arteries is caused by a build up of cholesterol and/or mineral salt deposits (commonly excess calcium) in the body. The former case is distinguishable from the latter in its appearance in the eye by a slightly yellow tint to the arc, but it is advisable to treat both possible causes to ensure that the arteries are cleansed.

In both of these cases it is important to take preventive measures.

Dietary guidelines

It is absolutely essential to change the diet in accordance with basic naturopathic preventive health care principles. In particular, the following points are most important.

Avoid salt   Table salt and foods to which salt has been added are best avoided. This is because sodium attracts and absorbs fluid; it therefore leads to excessive fluid in the blood vessels, and thereby puts unnecessary pressure on the cardio-vascular system. It is very much like trying to pour too much water down a blocked pipe; eventually some part of the piping will give way or burst.

Avoid mineral tablets   Mineral tablets may actually augment the condition, and in many cases will have caused or contributed to the onset of the condition in the first place. Mineral tablets are generally made synthetically and are not easily absorbed by the body. Consequently, it is not uncommon for the mineral salts to form deposits around the joints and in the artery walls.

It is far preferable to obtain minerals and other

187

nutrients from a wholesome balanced diet than from artificial tablets. When you feel that you need additional nutrients, get them in the form of freshly squeezed raw fruit and vegetable juices. Not only are these extremely nutritious, containing generous amounts of vitamins and minerals, which are easily absorbed and metabolised by the body, but they are also very cleansing as they contain the purest water, and this helps to dissolve toxic deposits in the body.

Avoid dairy foods   Reduce or avoid dairy foods, especially hard cheeses. All dairy products are high in saturated fats (especially hard cheeses). Furthermore, and contrary to popular belief, the calcium content in dairy foods is not easily assimilated by the body. Norway, for instance, has the largest consumption per capita of dairy foods in the world, and yet it also has the highest rate of osteoporosis (brittle bones) per capita.

One French ophthalmologist once commented to me that whenever he sees an arcus senilis in a patient's eyes he always says to them 'You love cheese, don't you', which invariably leaves the patients dumbstruck.

Avoid meats   All meats are best avoided, particularly red meats (including veal and pork); and as chicken has nearly as much cholesterol as red meats, poultry is not a healthy substitute and should be avoided as well.

The reason for this is that all meats are high in saturated fats and cholesterol, which clog up the arteries. Indeed, virtually every clinical and epidemiological study ever carried out on the subject confirms that meat is the single most important factor in heart-related diseases, as it raises the serum cholesterol levels in the bloodstream, which in turn helps to form the harmful deposits that line the arterial walls.

It is far better to aim to have a larger proportion of fresh fruits and vegetables in the diet, and to make use of the many vegetable and soya-based meat substitutes in order to ease the transition away from meat.

Additional advice

- Oats have been recommended by naturopaths for many years, but now it has been confirmed that the regular consumption of oats and oatbran can reduce blood cholesterol levels by up to 20 per cent.
- Lecithin is found in many foods and is a well-known emulsifier, helping to reduce cholesterol levels by breaking up accumulated fat deposits within the body. Lecithin granules can be added to meals, one teaspoon with each meal.
- Garlic has been shown to be effective in reducing cholesterol levels and cleansing the blood. Garlic has one-tenth the antibiotic strength of penicillin, and is renowned for its anti-coagulant qualities and its ability to lower blood pressure.
- Onions have similar properties to garlic. In one study one group was fed a fatty diet, another group a fatty diet plus onions. As expected the cholesterol levels in the volunteers shot up after being given the fatty foods, but it was found that by adding onions to the diet the tendency for the blood to clot was greatly reduced.
- Fresh fruits and raw vegetables, apart from providing easily assimilated nutrients, are also excellent blood cleansers.

For a fuller list of dietary guidelines to help reduce cholesterol levels in the blood *The Quick Cholesterol Clean-out* by Peter Cox and Peggy Brusseau is highly recommended.

Avoid creating emotional stress
Tension in the body will cause the arteries to narrow even further, and thereby increase the risk of a haemorrhage to an artery. Take time out during the day to slow down and unwind to prevent any tension building up.

Smoking – Don't!
This really goes without saying, and it is unfortunate that in our day and age it still has to be stressed. Smoking should be avoided as it constricts the capillaries and there-

fore further narrows the space through which the blood can flow. Smoking also increases the permeability of the artery walls, which means that more cholesterol deposits can stick to them.

In fact studies have shown that smoking actually increases the risk of heart-related diseases by up to 1,500 per cent. People who have an arcus senilis or, even worse, a cholesterol ring and who continue to smoke are therefore heading for serious trouble.

WEAK HEART TISSUE

Where the iris records a lacuna in the heart zone, it means that the heart tissue is inherently weak and requires strengthening. Diet and exercise consequently are very important.

Weight loss

It is very important that you lose weight. Every extra pound of excess fat means that the heart has to pump blood through an additional 200 miles of capillaries, not to mention the extra strain of carrying the excess weight. Try carrying a 3 lb sack of potatoes with you all day long and you will soon appreciate how heavy 3 lb of additional body weight actually is and how much extra effort it takes to carry it.

Other guidelines

- The diet should, of course, be kept low in foods containing high amounts of cholesterol and saturated fats (e.g. meats, cheeses, butter, chocolates, etc.), all of which put added strain on the heart and vascular system.
- Plenty of raw salads and vegetables will help keep the bloodstream pure; they cleanse the body and provide the vital nutrients in a form that can easily be assimilated by the tissues.
- If you smoke, stop. Not tomorrow, or next week, or next month; by then it may be too late. Smoking is a

killer and will hit fast where there is weak heart tissue.
- Herbal extract of hawthorn, in liquid form, is a traditional remedy for heart troubles and is excellent in cases of a weak or under-functioning heart (see page 48).
- Exercise. The heart, as we have mentioned, is only a muscle and, like any muscle in the body, if it is not exercised it will weaken.

TENDENCY TO VARICOSE VEINS

A tendency to varicose veins is seen in a net constitution and, more specifically, where there are lacunae in the blood zone at 6.00 in the iris.

The veins are vessels through which the blood travels back to the heart. Unlike the arteries, the flow of blood through the veins is dependent on the contraction of muscles around the veins; these squeeze the vessels and push the blood through them – the pumping action of the heart has little effect. Therefore once again we can see the importance of exercise to prevent another circulatory condition.

There are valves at intervals in the veins, and these prevent the backward flow of blood. If the tissue is weak, there will be a tendency for the valves to become incompetent and unable to function properly, and the veins then become varicosed, i.e. they balloon out as the blood accumulates in them.

Remedial advice
- Don't stand for long periods of time. Someone who has a tendency to develop varicose veins would be ill-advised to be in an occupation that involved standing for long periods, as the gravitational force puts further stress on the venous blood flow.
- Take up daily exercise. Daily exercise involving the leg muscles is essential to prevent the veins becoming varicosed.
- Reduce the saturated fats in your diet. Thick viscous

blood puts additional pressure on the valves and membranes of the veins; if you reduce the saturated fats in your diet you will tend to have thinner blood.

- Take regular hot and cold footbaths. These are an excellent aid to assisting the circulation all over the body, and particularly in the legs. The alternating hot and cold brings blood down to the feet and then pushes it back up again (see page 261).
- Sit with your feet up. Whenever possible, try sitting with your feet up to assist the flow of blood through the veins and back to the heart.
- Remedial massage physically moves the blood and lymph through the tissues. Whilst it is not advisable to have someone massage varicose veins directly, as a preventive measure a massage is of great benefit.

23
THE SKIN

The skin is the largest organ in the body and is often poorly neglected. It does far more than merely cover our bones and prevent us from drowning every time we have a bath. For example, the skin helps regulate body temperature and blood pressure; it manufactures vitamin D for use by the body; it protects the body against external germs.

But more importantly, the skin is one of the five major organs of elimination, and continually eliminates excess water, mineral salts and accumulated poisons from the body. In a comfortable room temperature, and without any strenuous exercise, the skin will excrete over half a pint of water during the day. And if strenuous exercise is carried out the skin can produce in excess of 14 pints (8 litres) of fluid during a day.

An inactive skin is often only a reflection of other internal troubles. For example, a sluggish and impure bloodstream and a general build up of toxaemia within the body will at some time affect the skin and lead to a variety of possible skin complaints. An inactive skin will also have serious implications for the rest of the body, because the other eliminating channels will be put under strain as they have to deal with the excess toxins.

Therefore if the rest of the body is to be kept healthy, the skin must be kept healthy; and, likewise, if the skin is to be kept fresh and healthy, the rest of the body must be kept healthy.

THE SCURF RIM

The scurf rim is the most common and easily detected iris sign reflecting the state of the skin. Furthermore, any discolourations of the skin zone of the iris will also be indicative of the condition of the skin in the related area. One man I saw had a very small whitish-yellow cloud in the upper back region in both irises. At the time he was not aware of anything in that area of his back, but on his way out he turned and pulled up his shirt to reveal a large sebaceous cyst in the middle of his upper back.

Improving elimination through the skin

Exercise Exercise, or, more particularly, exercising to the point of perspiration, not only improves general blood and lymph circulation but also stimulates elimination of toxins through the skin.

The importance of exercise and perspiration in the elimination of toxins from the body was highlighted by one young woman's fight against multiple sclerosis reported in *Prevention* magazine.

She had been suffering from slowly developing tingling sensations all over her body, followed by a deep fatigue, until it got to the point where it was an effort for her to walk even a few steps. However, being a fighter, she realised that drastic symptoms called for drastic action, so she dramatically changed her diet, cutting out all meats and glutenous foods (e.g. bread, cakes, and all wheat products) and replaced them with wholegrain rice, soya products, and with extra fruits and vegetables.

I felt stronger and stronger. So strong in fact, that I decided to run around the block. Much to my amazement, my legs held up. A few weeks later I even managed to jog around a running track. A quarter of a mile!

She did more and more exercise until, weeks later, whilst jogging around the ninth lap of the running track, she broke out into a sudden profuse sweat, something she could not recall having done for years. 'It was as if a dam had burst in my body', she said, and the more she sweated the better she felt. 'Perhaps I had been storing toxins for years and was finally releasing them', she surmised. 'Whatever the reason, my legs were springy, and while the tingling did not disappear, it retired into the background.' Eventually she was able to complete a half marathon successfully.

The story illustrates not just the importance of elimination of toxins through the skin but how, if the body is given the right conditions, it can 'heal' anything.

One word of warning, though. Do not exercise to the point of exhaustion, and always build up slowly. Do not put any undue strain on the heart; if you have any heart-related disorder consult your physician before taking up any form of exercise programme.

Steam baths and saunas   Saunas and steam baths again help the skin pores to open and sweat, thereby releasing toxins. However they can of themselves temporarily increase blood pressure, so if you are taking any medication to control blood pressure or have any cardio-vascular disorder, it is prudent to seek advice of your health practitioner before having a course of saunas or steam baths.

Skin brushing   Skin brushing is a quick and easy way of helping rid the skin of the dead cells that clog up the pores. Furthermore it also brings blood to nourish the skin tissues. A skin brush only takes a few minutes, and can be done virtually any time of the day, although it is particularly effective after drying the skin following a bath or shower. (For procedure, see pages 263–4).

Sunbathing   Sunshine is essential for all life on our planet, and is especially important for maintaining a healthy skin. Indeed many skin complaints, including acne, psoriasis and eczema, are greatly alleviated and improved by sunshine. Without sunshine the skin cannot produce vitamin D, which is required by the body in order to utilise calcium.

Unfortunately, however, sun exposure is also associated with melanoma, a highly lethal skin cancer, as well as with advanced signs of aging, such as dried, wrinkled skin. Therefore, sunbathing per se is not advised; or if one must do so, one should not lie out for more than half an hour at a time.

Of utmost importance before going out in the sun, whether for sunbathing or any other activity, is to apply a generous amount of sunscreen with a protective factor of at least 15, and preferably higher, to all exposed skin. This will not shut out the beneficial effects of the sun, but it will protect the skin from dangerous ultraviolet light.

PART III
FORESIGHT –
A PREVENTIVE
HEALTH LIFEPLAN

Health is created only by healthy living.

A.J. Jackson

Perhaps the time is not too far off when most of us will be able to care for our health by ourselves, and do so simply, using what nature freely offers. It must be recognized that everyone is capable of curing himself. No miracles are involved. It is inspiring to realize that each of us can test how free he is by practicing his own medicine in a simple manner.

Naboru Muramoto, *Healing Ourselves*

24
FOOD, DIET AND NUTRITION

Health and not disease is the true inheritance of life. Human creatures fail to realise facts which stare them in the face. We are made of what we eat, so if any organ becomes diseased, it generally means the food was wrong.

Major C. Fraser Mackenzie, *Health through Homeopathy*, 1944

We are what we eat – the food we eat today becomes part of us tomorrow. The nutrients we eat are not only utilised and stored in the body, but they actually become part of the body, forming the building materials of replenished tissue. For example, without sufficient calcium we develop brittle bones; without sufficient iron we become anaemic; without sufficient carbohydrate we have no energy; and without proteins we have no growth.

Good diet is therefore fundamental to creating and maintaining health. However, a healthy diet is not about obtaining certain quantities of different nutrients. Calcium, by itself, is not only useless but can be positively harmful, as any excess is deposited around joints, causing arthritic conditions, and on the arterial walls, causing arteriosclerosis (hardening of the arteries). To metabolise calcium, we need the other elements that are normally associated with it in nature – zinc, manganese, magnesium, etc. Furthermore, we need these other nutrients in the proportions found in nature. The same principle applies to the other known nutrients, and suggests that it might be better to avoid synthetically manufactured vitamin and mineral tablets and potions.

A healthy diet contains wholesome health-promoting foods – foods that are easily digested, and foods that contain and produce little waste. After the body has been nourished the waste has to be eliminated otherwise toxins will accumulate inside the body, and toxins accumulate in the stomach and intestines, foods eaten subsequently will not be digested efficiently. Therefore healthy digestion requires more than healthy food; it also needs healthy elimination.

To encourage good elimination of toxins from the body we first have to stop eating those foods which contain or create toxins, i.e. meats (including poultry) and fish, refined white flour products, refined sugars, artificial additives, colourings and preservatives, and hard cheeses. Some people find it a daunting and extremely difficult task to change their diet completely, although when faced with a clinically diagnosed disease such as arteriosclerosis (hardening of the arteries) or diabetes, we would have no option but to make immediate and often radical changes in our diet.

In preventive health care, the transition to a healthier diet need not be difficult or painful if you take one step at a time and gradually reduce the intake of these harmful foods rather than suddenly cut them out of the diet altogether.

Healthy digestion also depends upon healthy food combining. It is important not to combine certain foods that are difficult to digest simultaneously; as some foods hinder or obstruct the complete digestion of other foods, and this will lead to the creation of more toxins. These are called incompatible foods. The accompanying chart shows what foods are not compatible, e.g. high-protein foods should not be consumed with high-carbohydrate foods.

Listed below are some simple easy-to-follow guidelines on diet and nutrition. However, these are only guidelines and should be treated as such. Do not be too rigid with yourself at first. Where suggestions are new to you, start by trying to cut down and then slowly cut out altogether those things that are not recommended.

BASIC FOOD COMBINING CHART

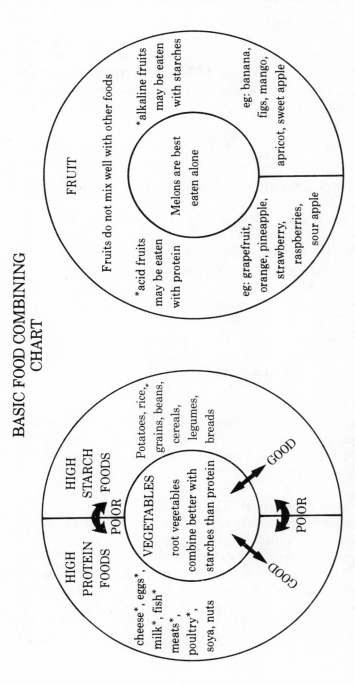

HIGH PROTEIN FOODS

cheese*, eggs*, milk*, fish*, meats*, poultry*, soya, nuts

HIGH STARCH FOODS

Potatoes, rice,* grains, beans, cereals, legumes, breads

VEGETABLES

root vegetables combine better with starches than protein

POOR

GOOD

GOOD

POOR

FRUIT

Fruits do not mix well with other foods

*acid fruits may be eaten with protein

*alkaline fruits may be eaten with starches

Melons are best eaten alone

eg: grapefruit, orange, pineapple, strawberry, raspberries, sour apple

eg: banana, figs, mango, apricot, sweet apple

* – Not recommended, listed for clarification only.
Drinking with or immediately after a meal dilutes the gastric juices.
It is better to eat fruits before other foods as they are then digested more quickly.

Also, remember that we are all different and that these guidelines are for a person with a normal healthy digestive system. Certain foods may not be beneficial to certain conditions; for example, if you have hyper-acidity in the stomach, citrus fruit would not be an ideal food as they are high in acids and would aggravate your condition.

THE DO's

Eat plenty of fruit, nuts, whole grains, and vegetables

These all contain vital nutrients – minerals, vitamins, essential fatty acids, enzymes, etc. in the right balance, as designed by nature. Raw fruits and vegetables are the most nourishing and easily digested; cooking destroys many nutrients, including vital enzymes and vitamins. In fact, studies have shown that health is best served when raw foods account for 50–75 per cent of the diet. (However, remember to wash thoroughly all foods that are not organically produced as the skins will contain toxic residues of pesticides and herbicides.)

Chew thoroughly

Digestion of carbohydrate foods begins in the mouth. Improperly chewed food will therefore lead to improperly digested food, producing wind, constipation and a host of other bowel disturbances.

Eat whole unrefined foods

Refined foods (e.g. white bread and white sugar products) have many essential nutrients taken out during their processing. To convert food into energy we need all of the elements that come with it in nature; without these the body will take the nutrients from its own tissues, thereby depleting it of resources. And don't be fooled by 'enriched' foods; these are refined foods from which many nutrients have been removed and then a few synthetic ones added.

Eat when relaxed

Negative emotions affect the digestive process. The digestive system works best when we are relaxed and comfortable.

Eat only when hungry, drink only when thirsty

Many people eat and drink, not because they are hungry or thirsty, but purely out of habit, frustration or boredom. Over-eating and over-drinking put unnecessary burdens on the digestive organs, which quickly become congested.

Drink water, fresh fruit and vegetable juices, herbals teas

All of these are refreshing, cleansing, and even therapeutic in their action within the body. But ordinary tap water contains mineral and chemical residues, including fluoride and chlorine, and has been found in some cases to be badly polluted with different strains of harmful bacteria. So it is best to drink only mineral, filtered or distilled water.

THE DON'Ts

Don't over-eat

Over-eating taxes the digestive system and takes blood to the abdomen, away from other areas of the body. The head is usually the first to suffer, and it is for this reason that over-eating often leaves you feeling lethargic and tired.

Don't eat when physically or emotionally exhausted

The digestive organs do not work efficiently when we are emotionally upset or physically tired.

Don't eat meats of any kind

The human body is simply not designed to digest flesh foods. We belong to the primate family, all of whom are herbivorous; even the great and mighty gorilla gets its strength solely from vegetation.

All clinical and epidemiological studies confirm that meat is a major factor in chronic degenerative diseases, from heart-related diseases to cancers. All meat, poultry and fish has in recent years become heavily contaminated with a plethora of toxic pollutants of alarming magnitudes, including hormones, antibiotics, nitrites and nitrates. Furthermore, animal meat is high in saturated fats, which are harmful to the cardio-vascular system. There are only two words of advice needed in respect to meat: Avoid it.

The effect of meat on the body is comprehensively documented in the book *Why You Don't Need Meat*, by Peter Cox – essential reading for anyone who is serious about their health.

Don't eat hard cheeses
Hard cheeses are very difficult to digest, being high in saturated fats and they create high levels of cholesterol in the blood.

Although dairy foods are rich in calcium, it is in a form perfect for calves but imperfect and not easily absorbed by humans. The calcium content in milk often tends to deposit in the arteries and in and around the joints, leading to arteriosclerosis (hardening of the arteries) and rheumatic/arthritic conditions.

Don't cook with aluminium cookware or foil
Aluminium is a soft metal which is associated with Alzheimer's disease, a form of senile dementia. It is very difficult to get out of the body once it has been ingested.

Don't consume artificial preservatives, colourings, flavourings
Don't eat any foods that contain any chemical additives. They all have unpleasant side effects, and no one really knows what their long-term results will be.

Don't eat a heavy meal in the evening

The body's metabolism is slow in the evening. 'Eat break-fast like a king, lunch like a prince and dinner like a pauper' is a very old saying, and clinical trials have proved the wisdom of it.

Don't drink coffee, tea, alcohol

All are stimulants and deplete the body of vital nutrients, create acidity and produce hypertension.

25
THE MEAT MYTH

A dead cow or sheep lying in a pasture is recognised as a carrion. The same sort of carcass dressed and hung up in a butcher's stall passes as food! Careful microscopic examination may show little or no difference between the fence corner carcass and the butcher shop carcass. Both are swarming with putrefaction.

Dr John Harvey Kellogg

The bacteria in meats are identical in character with those of manure and more numerous in some meats than in fresh manure.

A.W. Nelson, bacteriologist, Battle Creek Hospital and Sanatorium

Poultry should carry a government health warning.

Professor R. Lacey, microbiologist, Leeds University

Salmonella infects nearly 100 per cent of poultry.

Director of Central Public Health Laboratory

Poultry generally teems with harmful organisms that cause millions of food poisoning cases every year.

New Scientist, 3 September 1987

People in the main eat meat simply because they were raised on it by their parents and have acquired a taste for it. But just as palates are acquired, so they can be changed. Some may believe that it is perfectly natural and indeed healthy for humans to be carnivorous, and that we need animal protein for our health; but, as it will be shown

below, the contrary is true. Humans are by nature vegetarians, and meat eating is the major single causative
factor of most chronic degenerative diseases.

THE QUESTION OF PROTEIN

There has been no greater deception in the field of
nutrition than the idea that a high protein diet is necessary for optimum health and well-being.

Proteins are structural and functional compounds
found in all living organisms, both plant and animal. They
are made up from a range of about 20 amino acid building
blocks. The human body produces all these amino acids
itself save for 8 in an adult and 10 in a child. It is these 8
(10) amino acids that are called essential, for it is essential
that we get them from our diet. But whilst all of these
essential amino acids are found in meat, they are also
found in plant-based foods; cereals, nuts and legumes are
all high in essential amino acids.

The problem is not that people do not get enough
protein in their diet, but rather that they have far too
much. No one really knows the optimum amount of
protein that should be eaten – authorities differ, rec-
ommending between 39 grams and 110 grams per day,
depending upon age, sex, etc. The National Academy of
Sciences in the USA recommend 56 grams, but in their
literature have stated that we need only 30 grams. Why
the difference? When asked by the Robbins Research
Institute, they replied that they had met with a huge
public outcry when they had reduced the recommended
daily allowance from 80 grams to 56, so they felt that they
could not reduce it any further. However the 'huge public
outcry' was not from people like you and me, but from
those organisations with vested interests – yes, you've
guessed it, the meat industry.

Propaganda in this multi-million-dollar industry is no
less than outrageous. Consider a leaflet being circulated to
children in the UK, in which a government nutritionist
states that 'It is impossible to be healthy if you don't eat

meat'. Anyone with the slightest knowledge of nutrition knows that such a statement is simply wrong.

But what about the effects of excess protein? Meat contains high levels of uric acid, a waste product found in urine which puts stress on the kidneys and bladder, resulting in kidney stones. High levels of uric acid are also found in people suffering from leukaemia. The average piece of meat contains 14 grains (0.910 grams) of uric acid, but your body can only eliminate 8 grains (0.52 grams) in one day.

Therefore the problem facing most people is not whether they will get enough protein, or even whether they will get too much. The question is *how much* excess protein they will eat, and how much damage it will do to their body.

IS MEAT A NATURAL FOOD?

No physiologist would dispute with those who maintain that man ought to have a vegetable diet.

Dr Spencer Thompson, physiologist

Man belongs to the primate family, all members of which are complete vegetarians. It is a rare occurrence indeed to see a gorilla or a baboon dining off a carcass. And why should they? Their anatomy and physiology is simply not suited or designed to digest the dead flesh of another creature. Many of the world's populations and civilisations have remained vegetarian and are often healthier than their meat-eating counterparts. For instance, the Buddhist peoples in the Far East and indeed approximately 90 per cent of the population in India have been vegetarian for hundreds, and in some cases thousands, of years. The Hunza people of South America, also vegetarian, are renowned for their remarkable health and longevity. Scientists have also recorded how the (vegetarian) inhabitants of the Vilcabamba valley in Equador frequently live to be more than 100 years old and one person was recorded to be 142 years old.

Studies show time and time again that the major degenerative diseases of Western society including cancer, heart disease, and diabetes, hardly, if at all, affect vegetarian populations, and are practically unheard of in vegetarian cultures. The very first chapter of the Bible confirms that man was not designed to eat meat: 'Behold I give you every herb bearing seed and the fruit of the tree, for you it shall be as food' (Genesis 1,29).

Compare the anatomy and physiology of man with that of a typical herbivore (e.g. ape) and that of a typical carnivore (e.g. lion).

- Herbivores have jaws that move laterally and vertically, and teeth suited for grinding; carnivores' jaws move only vertically, and their teeth are suitable only for ripping.
- Carnivores have 15 times more hydrochloric acid in their stomachs than herbivores.
- Carnivores have on average only three feet of intestines, so that the flesh is expelled before it has time to putrefy. Herbivores have over 22 feet of intestines.

It does not take much common sense or knowledge of biology to see with whom we have more in common; it soon becomes clear that humans, by virtue of anatomy and physiology, were never intended to eat meat. Desmond Morris, the renowned anthropologist, confirmed this in his book *Manwatching*: 'In origin, man is a fruit-picking primate turned hunter'.

Meat is therefore not a part of our natural diet. It is not a healthy food and not part of a balanced diet. Dr Jay Hoffman explains:

When the animal is alive, the osmotic process in the colon keeps putrefactive bacteria from getting into the animal. When the animal is dead the osmotic process is gone and putrefactive bacteria swarm through the walls of the colon into the flesh.

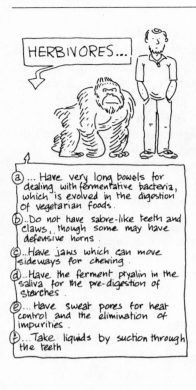

HERBIVORES...

(a) ... Have very long bowels for dealing with fermentative bacteria, which is evolved in the digestion of vegetarian foods.

(b) ..Do not have sabre-like teeth and claws, though some may have defensive horns.

(c) ..Have jaws which can move sideways for chewing.

(d) ...Have the ferment ptyalin in the saliva for the pre-digestion of starches.

(e) ... Have sweat pores for heat control and the elimination of impurities.

(f) ...Take liquids by suction through the teeth

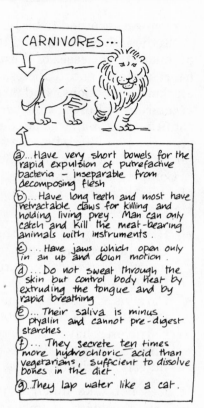

CARNIVORES...

(a) ...Have very short bowels for the rapid expulsion of putrefactive bacteria — inseparable from decomposing flesh

(b) ...Have long teeth and most have retractable claws for killing and holding living prey. Man can only catch and kill the meat-bearing animals with instruments.

(c) ... Have jaws which open only in an up and down motion.

(d) ...Do not sweat through the skin but control body heat by extruding the tongue and by rapid breathing

(e) ... Their saliva is minus ptyalin and cannot pre-digest starches

(f) ... They secrete ten times more hydrochloric acid than vegetarians, sufficient to dissolve bones in the diet.

(g) ..They lap water like a cat.

THE LEGACY OF INTENSIVE FARMING

Meat today contains far more than mere putrefactive bacteria. A four-ounce burger contains as much benzo-pyrene (a known carcinogen) as 600 cigarettes. It contains dangerously high levels of hormones, antibiotics, nitrates, nitrites and a plethora of other toxic chemicals that are fed or injected into the farmed animals.

Ninety-eight per cent of all the meat we eat comes from factory-farmed animals. These creatures are not only injected with toxic chemicals and growth promoters, they are also kept in buildings, never to graze in a field or feel the warmth of the sun, caged up so tightly that they are unable even to turn around. They are fed their own recycled excrement, together with the remains of unsaleable carcasses of their own species (i.e. they are forced to be cannibals).

Intensive farming practices also pollute the vegetation with fertilisers and pesticides, this being a necessary activity because so much vegetation is required to feed the huge animal populations in factory farms. So if the chemical pollution of a commercially grown carrot is calculated as one unit, the pollution level of a battery-reared chicken is over 10 million.

Apart from being morally abhorrent and offensive, this type of intensive farming rebounds on us, for as we have seen, the flesh of such creatures is highly toxic and carcinogenic (cancer-producing). In the past the choice has been between the savagery and butchery of carnivorous diet, with consequent ill-health, and the health-promoting natural diet of vegetarianism. But today the stakes are higher; the choice is between self-destruction and survival.

Mad Peoples' Disease

I believe, in years to come, that bovine spongiform encephalopathy (BSE) or 'mad cow disease' as it is better known, will cause a major epidemic amongst human populations. Several scientists have publicly declared that they have given up eating beef because of the disease. Among them are included Professor Philip James of the Rowett Research Institute in Scotland, and Professor Lacey of Leeds University Medical School. In fact Dr Dealler believes that people who eat infected meat have a fifty-fifty chance of contracting the disease. 'No-one,' he says, 'who knows enough about this subject would feed their daughter a beefburger.' Quoted from *Scottish Farmer* December 1990.

The disease affects the brains of cattle, and is caused by feeding the cattle with carcasses of dead sheep infected with a similar disease (scrapie). It's called 'mad cow disease' because it causes sudden brain damage and produces uncontrollable behavioural changes in these otherwise placid creatures. But is it surprising when most cattle in the UK, whether being reared for milk or beef, along with calves being fattened for veal, are fed animal bones, lymph glands, brains, other offal, skin, hair, gristle, and even recycled chicken excrement? Hardly a sensible diet for herbivorous creatures that would, by choice and nature, eat grass.

Doesn't the very idea of it seem repulsive? Yet we, in turn, eat their meat, drink their milk, and make medicines and vaccines from cattle blood serum. Scientists are beginning to question the safety as well as the morality of such practices.

One medical journalist reported: 'The question is: shouldn't it be called "mad peoples' disease"? For the scandal is not about a new mysterious infection sweeping through cattle but, I would suggest, a sickness that long ago swept through mankind. The reason we face any problem at all over BSE is that man has flouted the laws of nature.'

Whilst it may be true that many farmers are subject to a great deal of socio-economic pressures to produce cheap food, the modern farming practices are inexcusable; they are as abhorrent as they are shocking, and they create terrible dangers to human health and the environment at large.

The DES scandal

Diethylstilboestrol (DES) was the first synthesized oestrogen – developed in 1939 to prevent miscarriages. It was subsequently found not only to cause miscarriages (today it is used as a morning-after contraceptive pill), but also to cause a completely new type of cancer in the women who received it. And worse was to follow, for in later years it became evident that the children whose mothers had received DES also developed this new cancer, although the disease didn't develop in the child until he or she was between 15–25 years old.

Unfortunately, DES was introduced in farming when it was found that animals injected with the substance increased in weight by 30–40 per cent – more money with less effort in a shorter space of time. DES thus became the prototype for today's wide range of artificially prepared hormones that are injected into farm animals as growth promoters, and which are in the joints of meat that reach the meal table.

Meat and Cancer

All major clinical and epidemiological studies have shown that people eating a diet containing meats (including poultry) have a higher incidence of cancer. The higher the meat intake, the higher is the risk and incidence of cancer. For instance, one study carried out in Israel between 1949 and 1975 revealed that the number of deaths from cancers rose in proportion to the amount of animal fat, and in particular to the amount of meat, in the diet. Further studies undertaken in Alberta, Canada, and in Hawaii also revealed that the risk of contracting breast cancer increased in proportion to the amount of beef and pork in the diet. Studies done with over 49 different nationalities over 25-year periods all confirm that meat is the most significant single factor in the cause of all chronic degenerative disease.

In 1981 epidemiologists R. Doll and R. Peto concluded that diet is 'the largest single cause of all types of cancers (*The Causes of Cancer*, OUP), while in a comprehensive appraisal of the effects of meat on human health entitled *Why You Don't Need Meat*, Peter Cox cites countless studies that identify meat as a major factor in the causation of degenerative diseases. Listed below are a few of these studies:

- Women who consume the most animal fat in their diet double the risk of contracting ovarian cancer when compared with those who consume the least ('Dietary animal fat in relation to ovarian cancer risk', *Obstetrics and Gynecology*, June 1984).
- Men who consume animal products run four times the risk of contracting cancer of the prostate when compared to those who do not consume large quan-

tities ('Diet, obesity, and the risk of fatal prostate cancer', *American Journal of Epidemiology*, 1984).

- A significant risk factor in brain tumours in children is the consumption of nitrosamines [found in cured meats] by the mother ('N. nitroso compounds and childhood brain tumours', *Cancer Research*, 1982).
- A two-year study taking information from 37 nations concluded in 1966 that bowel cancers increased in direct proportion to the amount of meat in the diet ('Diet as an etiological factor in the development of cancers in the colon and the rectum', M.A. Howell, *Journal of Chronic Disease*, 1975).

MEAT AND HEART DISEASE

Today it is well accepted that meat adversely affects the cardio-vascular system. The high levels of saturated fats and cholesterol put stress on the heart and block the arteries. Indeed studies done in the UK, USA, Australia, Israel, Japan, Greece, Italy and Norway all confirm that meat (including poultry, which, contrary to popular belief, contains nearly as much cholesterol as beef) has a distinct and significant effect on heart disease. It is therefore hardly surprising that patients who have suffered heart and cardio-vascular disease are advised to reduce their intake of meat.

Conversely, evidence suggests that people who have high intakes of fresh fruits and vegetables have much less likelihood of suffering heart disease. Studies confirm conclusively that a reduced intake of meat leads to a reduced serum cholesterol level and reduced cardio-vascular disease.

THE NATURAL BALANCED DIET

The natural diet most suited to human beings and most

conducive to optimum health is a vegetarian diet. This contains all the nutrients we need, in their correct proportions and in a form that is easily assimilated, nourishing and cleansing.

Media propaganda has in the past labelled vegetarians as hippies and 'crackpots'. But who were those crackpots? Included in their number were: Voltaire, George Bernard Shaw, Ghandi, Socrates, Plato, Pythagorus, Leonardo da Vinci, Albert Schweitzer, Albert Einstein, Leo Tolstoy, Buddha, Isaac Newton, H.G. Wells, John Wesley, Percy B. Shelley, Plutarch, St Francis of Asissi, Henry David Thoreau, Benjamin Franklin – hardly a bunch of hippies.

Common sense alone suggests that if one is serious about preventive health care, meat should not form part of the diet. National and international clinical and epidemiological studies confirm that the diet best suited to man is a vegetarian diet.

- 'Vegetarian populations show decreased occurrence of heart disease, and colon and prostatic cancers. Heart disease and colon and prostatic cancer is directly proportional to meat and fat consumption' (J. Yaveloway of *Cancer Research*).
- 'Scientific evidence supports a positive relationship between the consumption of plant based foods and the prevention of certain diseases' (American Medical Association).

MEAT AND THE ENVIRONMENT

Meat in your diet does not just affect your health – it affects your world.

- Every minute of every day, an area of rain forest the size of 10 football pitches is destroyed, three-quarters of that destruction being solely to create grazing land for cattle to be reared for beefburgers. After a few years the land is left barren. Half a ton of tropical rainforest is destroyed to produce one half-pounder burger. An area of 9 square feet of one of the world's richest resources is lost forever, simply so that someone somewhere can have a beefburger.

- Half the world's population is starving, and yet 85 per cent of the world's grain is fed to factory-farmed animals. It takes 100 lb of cereal to produce 30 lb of meat, so for every meal containing meat, four people somewhere in the Third World will have to starve.

- There is only approximately 1 acre of arable land per person on the planet. On each acre can be produced enough vegetable and cereal produce to sustain between 30–60 people, but if the same acre of land is used to farm animals it will only feed two people.

- The less meat eaten, the fewer the animals that can be profitably reared; and the fewer the intensively reared animals, the less methane gas would be produced by flatulence. As the methane gas emitted from cattle is one of the largest contributors to the greenhouse effect, less meat eaten would mean a reduction in the greenhouse effect.

- If fewer animals were reared, there would be a reduction in the use of the toxic chemical fertilisers required to produce such vast quantities of cereal to feed the huge population of factory-farmed animals. Therefore if less meat were eaten this would reduce the destruction of the soil and the seepage of these chemical fertilisers which pollute the rivers at present.

- Less meat eaten would mean that fewer animals have to suffer the barbarism of a modern intensive farm, in which 98 per cent of all farmed animals 'live' in unimaginable conditions. Some animals never graze in an open field and never see the light of day, but instead are confined in a concrete building, chained up in cubicles so small that they cannot even turn round. They may be fed their own recycled excrement mixed with processed cereals and laced with antibiotics, hormone growth promoters and even the ends of unsaleable offal (the dead remains of their own species).

If we stopped eating meat, these factory farms could not exist. Some people ask 'Wouldn't the animals overrun us?' Of course they wouldn't. What happened before we had intensive farming? And what happens in those parts of the world today where there is no animal farming? Nature balances, and has done so not just for centuries but for millenia, long before factory farms were evolved.

What about 'organic meat'?

In addition to many health food shops and specialty grocery stores, more and more supermarkets are offering customers a choice of organic meats. These include poultry and the basic cuts of beef and pork. The animals are raised in generally humane conditions and consume only organically grown feed. The beef cattle generally graze on grass, rather than eat corn-based silage.

Organic meat is more expensive than other meat. This is because growers cannot raise as many animals as commercial farmers. For example, fewer cattle can graze per acre than can be fattened for market chained into stalls, row upon row in enormous barn. In addition, a field of organically grown grains for feeding chickens will experience more loss to insects and animals than one sprayed regularly with chemical pesticides.

Organic meat is clearly lower in chemical residues than factory farmed meat, and organic animal farming shows at least some concern for the welfare of animals and the environment. In this respect it must be considered preferable to factory farmed meat. However, I hope it has become plain from the reasons set out in this chapter that a meat-based diet, whether organic or inorganic, is totally contrary to natural and preventive health care principles and does not provide an answer to problems of ill-health or the larger environmental issues now facing us.

Peter Roberts, founder of Compassion in World Farming, an organization that has led the campaign against the dangerous and cruel intensive farming practices in the UK and throughout Europe, sums up the situation succinctly:

> As a vegetarian of 30 years' standing, meat plays no part
> in my personal life, and I would not be prepared to kill
> an animal or eat one. But when campaigning for the
> welfare of farm animals and appealing to the wider
> section of the community, 'organic' farming is often the
> first stepping stone for many people away from the
> barbaric modern animal farming practices because it
> incorporates a certain degree of welfare for farm
> animals and greater restrictions on the use of harmful
> drugs.

In short, organic meat is to be considered a preferable
alternative to factory-farmed meat, but for those people
who are serious about their health, their environment, the
starving people in the Third World, and the welfare of
animals, meat cannot remain part of their staple diet.

**The solution is simple. For the sake of your
health, and for the sake of the planet, leave meat out
of your diet.**

26
CHANGING YOUR DIET

> I think it could plausibly be argued that changes of diet are more important than changes of dynasty or even of religion.
>
> George Orwell, *The Road to Wigan Pier*, 1937

Changing your diet may turn out to be one of the most important changes you will ever make in your life. The food you eat affects not just your physical health but also your emotional well-being. For instance, refined foods deplete the body of vital elements and mineral nutrients such as zinc, iron and vitamin B, all of which are required for a healthy nervous system. By eating such foods we become more irritable, nervous, anxious and generally more susceptible to stressful situations.

High intakes of white sugar lead to unstable blood-sugar levels leading to hypoglycaemia and can cause the onset of diabetes. They are also associated with higher levels of irritability, and even violence. In fact studies with schoolchildren have shown that those children eating a diet high in sugars and refined foods have a much higher incidence of hyperactivity, reduced concentration and lower memory retention. Further studies in American and British prisons have also revealed that the number of violent outbreaks amongst prisoners may be substantially reduced when a diet rich in red meats, refined sugars and refined white flour products is replaced by a vegetarian wholefood diet.

But changing your diet may also have implications far beyond the simple betterment of your physical and emotional well-being. Change yourself and you will have an effect on those around you. Your tension and irritability can cause tension and irritability in your children, your partner and your work colleagues. Conversely, if you are calm and relaxed, you will have a calming and relaxing effect on those around you. If you are happier and healthier, then those around must also benefit. None of us lives in isolation.

So, change your diet and you begin to change the same world. We are all part of the world, and therefore when we change, the world changes. And the power of one individual to change the world for the better may extend far outside his or her own environment and community.

GETTING STARTED – A NEW WAY OF EATING

A thousand mile journey begins with the first step.

Lao Tse

Any change we make in our lives requires effort and determination, but with a little prior organisation the change to a healthier way of eating need not be difficult at all.

Keep it simple
In Chinese Taoist philosophy there is a saying that all things left in their original simplicity contain their natural power. The power is lost when the simplicity is changed. This principle applies to all aspects of life, but none more so than in food and diet. In the natural form, foods contain maximum power and life-giving elements. Cut a piece of fruit and within 20 minutes the vitamin C content has halved, due to oxidation. Cook it, and many of the vital enzymes necessary for digestion are lost, along with most of the vitamin content.

However, don't worry about trying to obtain so many grams of a certain vitamin or mineral. No other creature in the animal kingdom is concerned with vitamins and minerals, yet each creature eats according to its instincts and remains well nourished. For all our knowledge and wisdom in the field of nutrition, we suffer more diseases and disorders of the digestive system from poor quality foods than the whole of the animal kingdom put together.

We have become so obsessed with nutrients that we have lost the instinct of nutrition. If we are willing to return to the natural way of eating, and keep to the basic principles governed, not by laboratory experiments on rats, but by a fundamental understanding of nature and man's relationship to it, then we can't go wrong in our quest for a healthy diet. A healthy diet does not change with the fashion; it has been with us since the dawn of creation.

Remember that the bulk of the diet should be raw foods – fresh fruits, salads, vegetables – foods rich in pure, natural distilled water; cleansing, easily digested and packed with vital nutrients. All of the enzymes, minerals and vitamins are supplied in their correct proportions and are easily assimilated and absorbed into the blood stream. It is a mistake to think that we need high protein foods or concentrated carbohydrate foods for strength and energy. Remember, man belongs to the primate family, all of which are herbivorous. Gorillas have unmatched strength, yet live only off vegetation.

If you do cook fruits or vegetables, it should be as simply as possible – lightly steamed or baked with the minimum of added water. The easy way is to put the chopped vegetables into a saucepan and add a few table-spoons of water and a tablespoon of vegetable oil. Put the lid on, place on high heat, and within a few minutes the vegetables are fully cooked in the steam created by the water, while the oil forms a coating around the vegetables to prevent loss of nutrients.

Wholegrains provide carbohydrate – fuel for energy. To metabolise foods (i.e. to convert food into energy), there must also be present the nutrients – the minerals and vitamins – which are found in nature's unrefined whole foods. These nutrients are destroyed or extracted from refined foods (e.g. white breads, cakes made with white flour, sweets, chocolates and the like). Therefore when we eat refined foods, the body takes those nutrients from its own tissues in order to metabolise the food. Instead of nourishing us, it is easy to see how, in fact, eating those foods depletes the body of vital reserves. Try not to do it … or at least, not on a regular basis.

To cook wholegrains quickly and easily, simply use three parts water to one part grain. Bring the water and any seasoning (e.g. garlic, paprika, carraway seeds, and other herbs and spices for a natural flavouring) to the boil, add the grain and boil for five minutes. Then wrap the saucepan in towels or paper, and place in a box to keep it insulated. The grains will be fully cooked and perfectly fluffy within two to three hours, but can be left overnight.

Once you have cooked the grain, it can be used in a variety of ways:

- Add sautéed vegetables and a free-range egg and make into rissoles or burgers, to be grilled, roasted or baked.
- Add to soups and salads.
- As a base for savoury dishes such as risotto, curry, goulash etc.
- As a base for sweet dishes such as rice pudding.

Uncommon ingredients

Tofu Soya bean curd, an extremely versatile food. This is slightly alkaline, and a wonderful source of easily digested protein, containing all the essential amino acids. It can be flavoured for savoury dishes (e.g. chopped and cooked with a sauce and mixed vegetables), added to soups or stews, or mixed with a nut roast mixture. It can be marinated overnight in ginger or sweet and sour marinade, and eaten cold, grilled or roasted. Tofu is also wonderful in sweet dishes, whisked or mashed with soft fruit and honey, and can be used to make a delicious dairy-free 'cheesecake'.

Seaweed Seaweed has, ounce for ounce, over four times more calcium than cow's milk, over twice the amount of protein of a free range egg, and over ten times more iron than any meat, and yet remains low in calories. Sea vegetables, as seaweed should be called, are the richest food source available, containing generous amounts of virtually every known nutrient, including the so-called trace elements. Studies in Japan have shown that people who include sea vegetables as part of their daily diet enjoy a longer and healthier life.

Iodine is a difficult element to obtain from any other source but the sea, and is known particularly for its importance for a healthy thyroid (the gland that controls the body's metabolism); without iodine the thyroid becomes enlarged – a condition known as goitre. Sea vegetables are the most valuable source of iodine.

Despite the ever increasing pollution of the seas (which according to a recent Greenpeace study in the North Sea has led to one in four fish having visible cancerous growths), sea vegetables do not generally absorb pollutants, and they simply refuse to grow in areas where the pollution level is high. In fact, far from containing toxins, sea vegetables actually assist the body to eliminate radioactive and toxic metal pollutants. The high levels of alginic acid in sea vegetables bind with toxins in the body and help to enable their natural elimination.

Sea vegetables also help purify the blood through their strong alkalising effect, eliminating the high acidic wastes caused by the traditional Western diet. Furthermore, they help dissolve fats and mucus deposits that build up in the body.

Sea vegetables are usually sold in a dried form, and have to be soaked prior to preparation, the soaking time varying for the different types. There are many ways to prepare the vegetables; they can be put into soups and salads, cooked in a nut roast, deep fried and served as an hors d'oeuvre, or cooked in a light fragrant sauce and served as a side dish to a main course. In China Sze Tsu wrote in the sixth century that 'sea vegetables are a delicacy fit for the most honoured guest'.

Soy milk Soy milk is cheap and easy to make from soya beans, and is now widely available in many shops. It is less mucus-forming and more nutritious than dairy milk, and also free from the plethora of anitbiotics, hormones and bacteria commonly found in cow's milk.

Nut milks Nut milks are equally easy to make, almond milk being especially beneficial as it is highly alkaline. To make it, one cup of blanched almonds is liquefied with one quart of water, ½ a tablespoon of honey and a tablespoon of safflower oil.

The three seeds Sunflower, sesame and pumpkin seeds are all highly nutritious, containing proteins and essential fatty acids, vitamins and minerals. They may be eaten as a snack, roasted, added to savoury dishes/soups, or sprinkled on salads.

Apple cider vinegar Apple cider vinegar is a more alkaline alternative to the acid wine and malt vinegars.

PLANNING THE DAY

Breakfast like a king – the main meal of the day
Breakfast starts you off for the rest of the day. It is the time of the day when metabolism (the conversion of food into energy) is highest, for it is the time when your body most needs to be nourished.

- Fresh fruit salad
- Wholegrain cereals, e.g. muesli, oat/millet cereal with soy milk, creamed brown rice.
- Baked beans/mushrooms on toast.
- Freshly chopped green salad with avocado, and potato croquettes

Muesli The original muesli created by Dr Bircher-Benner bears very little resemblance to the so-called muesli one buys in the supermarkets and health stores today. Real muesli is made up of a tablespoon of rolled oats or other grain, a tablespoon of chopped nuts, and freshly chopped fruit with a little nut cream.

Lunch like a prince – the second main meal of the day

To be nutritious a meal need not be heavy. A heavy meal is one that takes a longer time to digest. Blood is then drawn to the stomach, away from other areas of the body, producing a feeling of lethargy and tiredness – not conducive to a productive afternoon's work. In contrast, a nutritious meal can also be light and easy to digest.

In a lunch box   Quick and easy things to put in a lunch box and take to work:

- Freshly chopped mixed salad with cider vinegar vinaigrette/lemon juice and cold pressed olive oil.
- Sprouted seed salad containing a mixture of sprouted alfalfa seeds, chickpeas, adzuki beans and mung beans.
- Fresh fruit.
- Wholemeal sandwiches, e.g. marmite and watercress, nut butters and cucumber, mushroom paté and green salad, banana and avocado – whatever takes your fancy. (Wholemeal bread may be replaced with rice cakes, oat cakes, rye-crisp, etc.)
- Cold vegetable burgers/cutlets/rissoles.

In a restaurant   There are normally plenty of nutritious foods on the menu:

- Vegetable soup (beware of the meat stocks, they are concentrated poison).
- Freshly chopped mixed salads.
- Steamed vegetables.
- Vegetable lasagne/risotto/burgers.
- Wholemeal pasta with a variety of sauces.
- Baked potato with butter.
- Vegetable curry.
- Vegetable shepherd's pie.

- Vegetable chilli.
- Stuffed cabbage rolls.

Supper like a pauper

Supper is best kept as a very light, easily digestible meal. In the evening metabolism is slow, and therefore heavy meals lead to unnecessary extra pounds gained in weight. A large meal also taxes the hormonal system, putting it to work, assisting in the digestive process, at a time when it would otherwise be slowing down. Furthermore, it places a burden on the nervous system, for the brain has to work most of the night sending messages to the stomach and intestines to secrete various digestive juices.

Ultimately regular heavy evening meals lead to a gain in weight, hormonal disturbance and nervous disorders. It is far better to follow the rest of nature and have a light meal.

- Soup and salad.
- Baked potato and ratatouille.
- Chinese stir-fry with marinated soya bean curd.
- Vegetable curry.
- Fresh fruit salad with soy cream and rye crispbread.

27
POSTURE AND EXERCISE

Exercise is essential to maintain the general health of the entire system.

Dr Herbert M. Shelton

The way we stand, the way we sit, the way we lie down, and the way we move and hold ourselves at all times constitutes what is referred to as posture. Ninety-nine per cent of the population have poor posture, caused purely by poor lifestyles; they simply do not have the energy to stand and sit upright and resist the pull of gravity. If everyone were to stand erect, sit upright and walk tall, the health of the population would be greatly improved.

It all begins in kindergarten and infant school. Children are trained from an early age to sit still, and are not given enough encouragement to stretch and exercise during school hours. In days gone by, during school holidays, children used to play outdoors; today, many merely sit in front of the TV. In a recent survey it was found that children spent on average three to five hours a day watching the television. The situation often gets worse in primary and secondary schools; one child who was brought to see me for chronic asthma attacks told me that at his school the children were only allowed two hours of physical exercise or games each week. Is it any wonder, then, that most of us have a poor posture and suffer from a host of health troubles that stem directly from it, such as reduced lung capacity, visceroptosis (prolapse of the abdomen, in which the abdominal muscles become flaccid and the internal organs drop) and poor circulation?

Exercise is crucial to sound health. An American

National Health Interview survey on the effects of regular exercise monitored over 7,000 people over a period of nine years, and found that men and women who didn't exercise were twice as likely to die early than those who did exercise. Similarly, a study conducted by Dr J. Dietrick at Cornell University Medical College found that people who are kept inactive develop general weakness, calcium loss from the bones and muscle atrophy. Yet another study, carried out by Dr Thomas Cureton, a former head of the Physical Fitness Laboratory at the University of Illinois, and involving over 50,000 participants, found that people who are unfit consequently suffer from poor circulation and loss of energy, and 'become introverted, with tendencies to anxiety, over-sensitiveness, and mental fatigue'.

Our posture is affected by the condition of the muscles, which hold the bones together. The strength of the muscles is in turn determined by nutrition, exercise and our general lifestyle, including our emotions.

Improvement will only come about if we change, and the place to start is to notice the types of foods you are eating, the types of exercises you are doing, your daily routines and your general emotional state.

NUTRITION

An imbalanced diet leads to imbalanced posture. A lack of absorbable nutrients will result in poorly nourished and weak tissues, which become physically unable to maintain a sound posture. Refined foods rob the body's tissues of vital nutrients, and much needed mineral reserves stored in the bones and muscle tissues become depleted.

What is needed is for good bone health, for instance, is a balanced wholefood diet, rich in green leafy vegetables, to ensure an adequate supply of absorbable calcium, magnesium and other important minerals. When the body is depleted of its calcium reserves, the bones become brittle and the general posture deteriorates.

Poor posture will also, in its turn, create poor digestion, because, when the body is slouched, the abdomen and the organs within it become cramped. The stomach and intestines, the spleen, the liver and the pancreas are all affected. The blood supply to and from them is hindered and consequently they begin to malfunction, as a direct result of the postural disturbance.

DAILY ROUTINES

Daily routines and habits gradually form our posture. The particular muscle groups that are used over and over again slowly become too strong for their opposing muscle groups.

At a physical therapy seminar my own posture was examined, in order to illustrate the effects our daily routines have on the body structure. My left shoulder blade was found to be approximately 1½ inches higher than my right shoulder blade. I had no pains whatsoever, but the distortion between the left and right shoulders was clearly evident. I was then asked if I spent much of my day on the telephone, and then it hit me – I spent virtually my entire day on the phone, which was held between my left shoulder and my ear.

Fortunately in my case the situation had not reached the symptom level and I was able to take remedial action, but other people are not so lucky. One man visited my clinic with a constant ache in the left side of his lower back. His left iris showed an accumulation of toxic wastes in that region of the body, but despite regular treatments the pain persisted, albeit in reduced intensity. It was only when I saw him coming into the clinic, carrying a brief-case, that the cause of the problem dawned on me. It was a large briefcase, and particularly heavy. I asked him if he always carried it in his left hand, to which he replied that he did. How often did he have to carry it? 'Several hours each day.' By carrying it in his left hand every day he was continually straining the left side of his lower back. As soon as he tried alternating the briefcase between his left and right hands, his back pain disappeared.

EXERCISE

Exercise is essential for muscular strength. In fact if you were to bind up one of your arms for a few days and then compare it to the other, you would find that, even in that short space of time, the bound muscles would have already started to atrophy and weaken.

To maintain a balanced posture, we therefore need balanced exercise. Many types of exercise and sport tend to be one-sided, and therefore distort the muscle balance and posture. Tennis and golf are good examples of one-sided sports that can dramatically affect your posture, unless preventive measures are taken to counter the imbalance. In tennis, for instance, one tends to be continually leaning slightly backwards and to the left when serving. Therefore it is sensible at times during the game to stretch the torso in the opposite direction, and thus maintain a balance.

Working out in a gym is perhaps the most notorious type of exercise taken these days as it can cause chronic distortion of the muscle balance and posture. All muscles work in pairs – the biceps and the triceps in the upper arm, the lower back and the abdomen, the quadriceps and the hamstrings in the legs, all work with each other. When one is flexed the other is relaxed. But what many people tend to neglect is that there is a natural equilibrium or balance of strength between two antagonistic muscles. And in many cases body building can disrupt that equilibrium.

A good example of such disruption can occur in the quadriceps on the front of the upper leg and the hamstrings behind. The quadriceps are, in their natural state, approximately 30 per cent stronger than the hamstrings. Therefore, when lifting weights, it is important either to make sure that 30 per cent more weight is given to the quadriceps or, alternatively, if the same weights are used, to ensure that 30 per cent more repetitions are done with the quadriceps. Most people, however, simply lift the same weights the same number of times with both muscle groups; over the weeks the muscles therefore lose their balance, and this is followed later by troublesome knee joints. It is therefore always advisable to seek professional instruction before using any body building/gym equipment. All gyms should have qualified instructors at hand. Don't try to do it yourself without getting advice first.

Try to see how your sport may be affecting your posture. If you always lean, stretch or push in one direction, stretch yourself intermittently in the opposite direction. Do regular full-body stretching exercises, from your head to your toes, to keep the joints and muscles flexible.

POSTURE AND EMOTIONS

Exercise and posture do not just affect the physical body; they have just as powerful an impact on the mind. This fact was highlighted at the turn of the century by F.M. Alexander in the development of his postural re-education technique known as the Alexander technique. The influence of exercise and posture on the emotions is now becoming more and more acknowledged and supported by clinical research.

So, although it sounds perhaps far fetched at first, the way we move, the way we hold ourselves, may actually create our emotional states. Anthony Robbins, in his book *Unlimited Power* states: 'If you change your physiology – that is your posture, your breathing patterns, your muscular tension, your tonality – you instantly change your internal representations and your (emotional) state'. A strong statement, but think about it for a moment.

If I told you that there was a 'depressed' man sitting in front of me, would you have any idea what his posture might be? Most people would imagine the man to be slumped, shoulders bowed forwards, head looking down, with a shallow breathing pattern and flaccid facial muscles. After all, have you ever seen a depressed person walking tall, with shoulders held back and head held high?

I doubt it, because it is extremely difficult to be depressed whilst maintaining that posture. Even people suffering from so-called manic depression are unable to be in a state of depression whilst maintaining such a positive posture, particularly when they put a smile on their face.

Therefore the first step towards changing your emotions is to change your posture.

A BETTER POSTURE EXERCISE PROGRAMME

The following series of exercises is designed to improve and correct your posture. They will help improve blood circulation, increase joint mobility and tone up the major muscle groups in the body, and so promote health. The exercises will only take between 15 and 20 minutes of your time each day – time well spent, because it will provide the basis for correcting posture and building up the musculature of the body, and thereby preventing posture - related illnesses.

Wear loose comfortable clothing when doing these exercises, so that movement is not restricted. The exercises should be done slowly and gently, definitely not fast and jerky. It is, of course, better to do them outdoors in a park or your back garden; if this is not possible, use a well-ventilated room, to provide as much fresh air as possible.

Proper breathing is essential if you are to get full benefit from any exercise. We can survive for weeks without food, and for days without water, but if we are deprived of oxygen for any longer than three minutes, our brain is quickly damaged or dies. So concentrate on breathing out on the exertion part of an exercise, as this will ensure that the tissues are well oxygenated.

Doing these stretching exercises regularly will quickly bring great dividends, which will be noticeable after a few weeks. Action brings power, and inaction brings debility, so choose power.

Eyes
● Look up as far as possible, and then down.

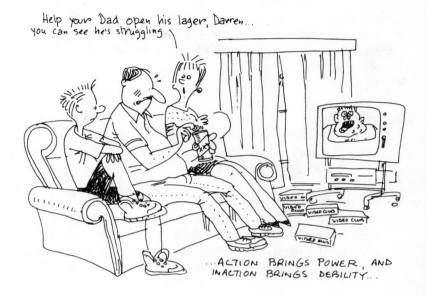

Help your Dad open his lager, Darren...
you can see he's struggling.

...ACTION BRINGS POWER, AND
INACTION BRINGS DEBILITY...

- Look to the right and then to the left.
- Repeat seven times.

Face and mouth
- Open your mouth as wide as possible.
- Then push the lips together.
- Yawn as widely as possible.
- Repeat seven times.

Neck and shoulders
- Stretch your neck from side to side, up and down.
- Try to move your head sideways down to your shoulder.
- Repeat seven times.

Upper back
- Clasping your hands together, stretch both arms upwards above your head as far as possible.
- Then stretch them outwards in front of your chest, again as far as possible.
- Repeat seven times.

Spine (side)
- Put your left arm on your left hip, with your right arm raised above your head, and slowly bend to the left.
- Reverse sides.
- Repeat seven times.

Spine (central)
- Lie on the floor, face upwards, and bring both knees up to your chest. Clasp your arms around the knees and rock backwards and forwards for approximately 45 seconds.
- On all fours, spreading your weight evenly between your knees and your hands, arch the spine upwards with your head facing the floor whilst exhaling. Then reverse the arch, with your head trying to look as far upwards as possible. Repeat seven times.

Spine (lower)
- Lie face upwards with your legs at 45 degrees but both feet remaining on the floor, about shoulder-width apart. Using the abdominal and lower back muscles, press the lower back against the floor whilst exhaling. (You should feel the abdominal muscles tense during this exercise.) Repeat seven times.
- Do the same as above, except this time straighten the right leg, moving the foot along the floor, as you push the lower back down. Then straighten the left leg whilst pulling the right leg upwards to its original position. Repeat seven times.

Abdomen
- Stand up, bend slightly forwards and rest your hands on your thighs for support.
- Breath out as fast as possible, then pull in your tummy muscles in quick repetition seven times.
- Repeat seven times.

Hips
- Stand with your feet shoulder-width apart, and slowly

bend forwards, arms stretched and hands held together.
- Move your trunk clockwise in as large a circular motion as possible.
- Repeat seven times.
- Then do the same movement anti-clockwise.

Thighs and legs
- Stand with your back against a wall, your feet shoulder-width apart.
- Gradually bend your knees whilst lowering yourself into a semi-squatting position.
- Hold this position for 30 seconds.
- Gradually increase over the following weeks to one or two minutes.

Feet and ankles
- Move one foot in a wide circular motion.
- Then stretch the foot up and down.
- Repeat seven times.
- Then do the other foot.

THE FIVE-MINUTE OFFICE WORKOUT

The five-minute office workout is a series of exercises specifically designed to prevent chronic neck and back disorders that result from working in an office environment. The exercises combat the effects of postural strain caused by typical office work, from simply sitting in meetings all day to typing, and even from being on the phone. The exercises stretch and help recondition all of the main muscle groups centring around the neck and the whole spinal column which are commonly distorted by sedentary occupations.

The whole workout is easy to do, as well as being quick and efficient. They may be done anywhere and will take no more time to do than the name suggests – five minutes. If done twice each day during the morning and afternoon it will help prevent the build up of chronic muscle fatigue and tension, leaving you feeling fresher and more relaxed.

How to do the exercises   Each exercise is a slow sustained stretch but *do not* stretch to the point of pain. Take the stretch to the point of mild tension and hold it there for 10 seconds. Then take it a little further and continue seven times. The breathing pattern is very important. Always inhale before the stretch and after the stretch, and exhale during the stretch.

The work-out   Commence by sitting in a relaxed position:

1. Drop your head forward and to one side until you feel the opposite side of the neck stretch. Repeat with the other side.
2. Side bend your head bringing your ear to your shoulder, but try not to raise your shoulder up towards your ear. Let the ear go to the shoulder. Again take it to the stretch, hold and continue as directed above. Repeat with the other side.
3. Look slowly to the left until you feel a stretch, and hold. Repeat seven times and then do the same only looking to the right.
4. Interlace fingers and stretch arms upwards above your head.
5. Keeping fingers interlaced, straighten your arms out in front of you with your palms facing outwards.
6. Still keeping fingers interlaced, put arms above your head and move the arms to the left, and hold. Then repeat to the right side.
7. Put the right arm behind the right side of your neck and gently push the right elbow with your left hand. Repeat with the other arm.
8. Pull your left elbow towards your right shoulder. Repeat pulling your right elbow to your left shoulder.
9. Hold both arms out at the side at shoulder level and pull them backwards.
10. Gently lean forward on your chair trying to touch your chest to your knees.

11. Place both hands on a wall or cabinet about chest level standing one pace away from the wall or cabinet with feet shoulder width apart. Then, keeping your hands at the same level, let your torso drop down stretching your upper back.

12. Sitting on the floor, keep your left leg straight and bend your right leg placing your right foot on the outside of your left knee. Then using your right arm as a lever against your right knee twist your upper body to the left trying to look as far behind you as you can. Repeat on the other side.

ISOMETRIC EXERCISES

Isometric literally means 'of the same length', and therefore exercise in which the muscle exerts pressure but remains the same length is called 'isometric exercise'. For instance, if both hands are clasped and pushing with equal force in opposite directions, the muscles in both arms tense but do not change in size, unlike lifting a bar bell when the muscle contracts in size as more pressure is exerted. The exercise employs maximum effort against resistance for a few seconds and is followed by complete relaxation of the muscle, and then repeated several times. Always exhale when exerting pressure to oxygenate the tissues fully. Much research has been carried out on isometric exercise in recent years and it has been found that in the case of healthy persons, brief isometric exercise of only 2-5 seconds (10 times) performed daily will produce an increase in strength.

28
THE MIND
& SPIRIT

A man is as he is in his heart.

Proverbs

In spite of all controversy, by proven and established facts, even at the present day ... except for the mind, the body would be a piece of mechanism.

Professor Alexander Erskine

The seed of all dis-ease begins in the mind. In fact, everything begins in the mind whether it be our desire to eat, or the will to do something or go somewhere. It all starts in the mind because it is the mind that controls the body. Our chosen thoughts create our emotions and drive our actions, but those same thoughts also affect and reflect the condition of the body. For when the mind is weak, the body is weak; when the mind is tense, the body is tense; but when the mind is strong, the body is healthy.

We have already seen in earlier chapters how specific emotions may affect specific organs. If the condition of the mind is neglected, health will rarely be maintained because failure to look after and strengthen the mind is like trying to build a house on sand. The mind is the very foundation of health. If we eat the best foods in the world they will do us very little good if we are in emotional turmoil because the digestive system will not function efficiently in periods of emotional distress.

STRESSES AND STRAINS

Stress is a killer, of that there is no doubt. It plays a part in virtually every degenerative disease known to the Western world. All around us we hear of the horrors that stress wreaks on our health. But stress is only a tension or pressure. Try to imagine your muscles if you never put them under some tension, if you never did any exercise. What would happen? The muscles would atrophy and degenerate; they would waste away.

Just as physical tension is necessary for physical growth and developing muscular strength, so too is emotional tension necessary for emotional maturity and for developing strength of character and spirit. Stress therefore is not our enemy; it alerts us to danger and is our best friend. Any disease, damage, disruption, call it what you will, is never created by stress. It is our reaction to the stress, whether physical or emotional, that is for the most part destructive. Being late for work simply cannot harm you, but allowing yourself to get agitated as a result will.

- Stressful situations cannot harm us, but our chosen reactions can.

THE DIFFERENCE THAT MAKES THE DIFFERENCE – ATTITUDE

There is only one important difference between those people who are happy and successful, and those people who are unhappy and unsuccessful, and that is the way they think – their attitude to life. It is purely the way we think that shapes our actions, and our actions shape our lives.

Have you ever wondered why it is that two people can experience the same blessings, or suffer the same or similar tragedies in life, and yet both react entirely differently? Ask two people to look up at the sky and tell you what they see. One may see patches of blue sky and sun, whereas the other sees only clouds. It is the same sky, but the two people have different perceptions of it.

People who rise above situations and overcome seemingly impossible hurdles in life generally share a common belief – that everything that happens in life, even the most dire of circumstances, happens for a reason, and can be used for our benefit.

There are many examples: Mike Brace lost his sight at the age of ten when a glass bottle containing fireworks exploded in his face, but he overcame his blindness to become a champion cross country skier and social worker.

W.J. Mitchell had a motor cycle accident that resulted in major and disfiguring burns to most of his body. His fingers were burned to a stubble and pain killing drugs had no effect. Several years later and after building up a major company and becoming a millionaire, Mitchell had yet another accident which left him paralysed from the waist down and shortly afterwards his wife left him. Yet Mitchell refused to give up. He founded his own radio station, ran for mayor and, despite his physical deformities, even attracted the woman of his dreams. He remains a source of possibility and inspiration to everyone who has heard of him.

Winston Churchill started out with a speech impediment and was looked upon as a poor pupil at school, yet at the age of 24 he won the Nobel prize and became known as one of the greatest orators of the twentieth century.

Thomas Edison was expelled from school and later given the sack from his first job, yet he went on to become the foremost inventor of our times.

Julio Iglesias had a severe accident which left him hospitalised. Yet it was during his stay in hospital that he decided to learn to play the guitar and to sing, and he went on to become the world's best selling recording artist.

One of the best examples of how human tragedy can be turned into triumph is Abraham Lincoln who became bankrupt at 31, and lost an election race at 32. His sweetheart died when he was 35 and he had a nervous breakdown at 36. He lost election races when he was 43, 46 and 48. He lost a senatorial race at 55, and failed to be elected vice-president at 56, yet at 60 years old he became President of the United States and is remembered as one of the greatest leaders in world history.

The truth is that many of the greatest of human achievements have been preceded by tragedies. The list of people who have turned seemingly impossible adversity into gain is endless and even includes people born with the most terrible congenital birth defects such as Christie Brown (author of *My Left Foot*), and Pete Strudwick, born with no hands or feet who went on to become a marathon runner.

- The blacker the cloud, the brighter the silver lining, if we are only willing to see it.

AGAINST ALL ODDS

Even suffering brings with it an opportunity of growth, the chance to rise to the challenge; pain can be an opportunity to change for the better and become stronger. Those situations that seem hopeless offer the chance to grow through suffering into a better, stronger you.

I remember how my eyes were opened to this fact after seeing a play called *Who's Life Is it Anyway?* The play is about a man who has had an accident which leaves him a quadriplegic – paralysed from the neck down. After the accident he decides that he no longer desires to live and through the courts he fights for the right to end his life by having his life support machine turned off. After the play was over a discussion ensued, led by a panel of four men, of whom two had become quadriplegic, one was paraplegic (paralysed from the waist down), and the fourth was a clinical psychologist. All three disabled men had suffered accidents which had led to their conditions, yet all three men emphatically stated that their lives were more meaningful and more fulfilled than they had been before-hand. They had achieved more with their disabilities than they had without them, because they had suddenly been confronted with despairing challenges that they had conquered.

- Greater challenges bring greater rewards.

THE MEANING OF YOUR LIFE

In his book *Man's Search For Meaning* Dr Victor Frankl, a psychiatrist who was incarcerated in a Nazi extermination camp during the Second World War, tells of how men existing in some of the most horrific conditions ever known managed to overcome and rise above their situation. Dr Frankl noticed that many men were choosing to die rather than face a seemingly endless hell on earth. Yet he found that mere words could be placed into a single sentence and could restore to those men a will to fight on; just one sentence could give renewed meaning to a man's life: 'What is the first thing you are going to do when you get out of here?' One man said he would find his wife, another would finish his thesis. Suddenly each man could find a purpose in his suffering, and a reason to live.

This is the difference between those people who overcome situations and those who collapse and crumble when faced with adversity. The winners give a meaning and a purpose to their situation; they choose to put a positive gloss on each event in their life. Everything, whether outwardly good or bad in appearance, is considered by them as having value and to be used for their benefit.

Nothing in your life has meaning except the meaning you choose to give it. Every coin has two sides. For example, you walk into work and are promptly given the sack. This could mean the end of your career and the start of depression; or it could mean that you have been given an opportunity to make a change of direction in life, to do better and bigger things. Similarly, if you experience a broken relationship it could mean that you have failed, that you're not worthy or capable of loving, that you are ugly, and that you have lost the best person you are ever likely to have a relationship with. Alternatively, you could choose to say it means that the two of you were perhaps not well suited, that you deserve someone who will appreciate you, that you are free to live as you want to live, and that it means there is now room for someone much better to enter your life.

It all hangs on what meaning we decide to attach to a particular event. So why not choose to give your life and the events within it a positive meaning rather than a negative one? 'There is nothing good nor bad, except he that makes it so' – so wrote Shakespeare.

There is an old story of a farmer in a little village in China. He owned a stallion, and one day it broke loose and fled from the farm. 'How terrible', the neighbours exclaimed, 'to have lost your prize stallion'. But the farmer replied 'Maybe bad, maybe good'.

Two days later the stallion returned with three mares. 'How wonderful', exclaimed the neighbours, but the farmer continued 'Maybe good, maybe bad'.

The next day one of the mares kicked the farmer's son and caused him to be hospitalised. 'How terrible', muttered the neighbours. But again the farmer continued, 'Maybe bad, maybe good'.

The following day war broke out, and all young men were conscripted, except for the farmer's son who lay in hospital. 'What luck' exclaimed the neighbours. But the farmer knew: 'Maybe good, maybe bad' . . .

The story teaches that things are not always as they may at first seem. And if we could understand the fine tapestry of life, we might just see how the intricate pattern of events was woven for our benefit.

- All things that happen in life can only serve for your betterment, bringing you closer to your goal, unless you choose to put a different meaning on them.

PROBLEM SOLVING

Problem solving is all a matter of how we choose to think in a given situation; all you have to do is ask yourself 'What can I do to remedy the situation?' If there is something you can do, do it. Rise to the challenge and take the opportunity to see how effective you can be. And if nothing can be done, simply relax. Remind yourself that 100 years from now it probably won't make the slightest bit of differ-

ence. As Tony Robbins put it in his book *Unlimited Power*: 'Here's a two step formula for dealing with stress
- Don't sweat the small stuff.
- Remember it's all small stuff!'

There is nothing frightening about stress. It is simply a way to self growth. However, that is not to say that there are times to fight and hold on, and times to walk away and let go.

Compare it with physical stress again. If you tried to run a marathon tomorrow, chances are you wouldn't make it, and if you did you might injure yourself in the process. But if you prepared yourself by training for several months you would stand a much better chance of making it past the finishing post. The same is true for mental stress. Take only what you can handle at any particular time, and the next day you will be able to tackle a larger load.

This is beautifully summarised by a prayer written by the Reverend Robert Schuller: 'Lord grant me the guidance to know when to hold on, and when to let go, and the grace to make the right decision with dignity.'

- There is no problem bigger than you.

IN SEARCH OF HAPPINESS

Too often we are conditioned to think that happiness is dependent upon external things. We think that happiness is something that we will miraculously be given or find once we achieve something or obtain something. We even tend to put conditions on our happiness: 'I'll be happy when I have a sports car', 'I'll be happy when I pass my exams', 'I'll be happy when I have a girlfriend ... or boyfriend ... or my own home.'

But when we achieve those things we suddenly realise that we must have been mistaken, because we still don't feel really happy. So we go about setting new conditions to determine when we really will be happy; fame, fortune, holidays, jobs, relationships, all become images of what we think brings happiness.

Yet if fame and fortune bring happiness, why is it that so many celebrities become alcoholics and drug addicts? If money brings happiness, why is it that the class of people who smile and laugh least are millionaires? Happiness and fulfillment are not determined by circumstances. It does not matter if you win a million-dollar lottery or lose your job. What does matter is how you react to the circumstances, rather than the circumstances themselves. The question is whether you are a master or a slave to circumstance, whether you can take responsibility for your life. With the right attitude, negative can be turned into positive; everything seen as for your betterment is for your betterment.

Eventually we realise that happiness is not what we have or what is about us; it is who we are and what is within us. Happiness is really only a state of mind and is created by focusing on the good things rather than the not-so-good. It is an attitude of gratitude. Whatever happens, if you are still alive you still have the greatest gift of all, because being alive but penniless is better than being dead and having a large bank account. Whatever our circumstances if we are alive, we have a reason to be happy. All it takes is a belief that your life can make a difference; that your life has a meaning, and a purpose. And nothing, but nothing, can prevent you from fulfilling that purpose!

- Happiness is a state of mind we can create at any moment simply by focusing on the positive rather than the negative, and by asking 'what's great'? or 'what could be great?' Gratitude creates a happy attitude.

FAITH

Very often we do not know what it is that brings about the recovery of the patient. I am sure that often it is a faith which is a most important factor.

Professor C.E. Forkner MD, Former President of the
New York Cancer Society

Faith is fundamental to life, for without faith people live in fear. By faith, I do not just refer to a faith in a God, or in a supernatural force, but a belief and trust in life. A belief that our lives are not part of some random selection, but the fulfillment of purpose.

A faith in a higher power or force is a prerequisite for faith in life, yet many people do not believe in anything. You need only look at the human body and indeed the whole of nature to see perfect design, and where there is design, is there not also a 'designer'? To think that there is no God, or higher 'power' or 'force', call it what you will, is like suggesting that the QE2 was formed over millions of years by bits of wood and plastic and metals slowly forging themselves into the magnificent ship we see today. It is like suggesting that the *Oxford English Dictionary* came about by a sudden explosion.

Albert Einstein once created a miniature clockwork planetarium and showed it to his atheist friends who were aghast at the machine and asked how he made it. Einstein replied that he didn't make it but it just came together of its own accord. 'But surely sir, it is a clockwork machine, someone must have made it?' they insisted. 'Why is it that you know that this fragile little machine which has to be continually wound up has been created, and yet it is only a poor imitation of the real thing in the heavens above of which you insist there was no creator?'

Faith leads to trust, and trust leads to peace of mind. It lightens the burdens of life and releases a force that can overcome seemingly insuperable odds. Men and women survived through concentration camps on meagre amounts of the poorest quality foods (and I use the term 'food' in its loosest sense) scientists have shown in clinical tests to be so inadequate that human life could not be sustained on them. Yet nevertheless people managed to survive and prove that life is more than molecules and chemicals. It is, at its truest level, a spirit or force that can overcome anything and has the power to move mountains.

Studies have shown again and again that a faith in a God, force or higher power is one of the most crucial factors in overcoming any disease. Often, and particularly in chronic and degenerative diseases, faith is the primary factor in a patient's recovery. Likewise it must also be considered a vital factor in maintaining health. Faith that no obstacle put in your way is big enough to stop you, that there is no gap that cannot be bridged, and no wall that cannot be broken down.

- **With faith, there is no situation you cannot face and overcome.**

29
LAUGHTER – THE BEST MEDICINE

A merry heart does good like a medicine.

Proverbs

There is no medicine in the world that can even remotely be compared with laughter. A good belly laugh eases the mind, alleviates pain, opens up the lungs, and massages the abdominal organs better than any masseur could possibly achieve. Voltaire wrote that 'The art of medicine lies in amusing the patient while nature will take its course', and never were truer words spoken.

The miraculous effects of laughter as a form of therapy were highlighted by Norman Cousins in his book *Anatomy of an Illness*. Cousins wrote of how he 'cured' himself of a crippling arthritic disease that had caused him to be bedridden with pain and which his doctors had told him was virtually irreversible, with less than a one in 500 chance of recovery. How did he do it?

In searing pain, Mr Cousins discharged himself from his hospital bed and took himself off the prescribed pain-killers, which he felt were making him feel worse. He then took to watching films and video tapes that made him laugh, most notably the Marx Brothers films. To his amazement, he found that the laughter alleviated the pain for several hours at a time. Coupled with dietary changes and vitamin supplements, he made a full recovery.

No one knows exactly why laughter has such a thera-peutic effect on the body, but it doesn't take much thought to understand the various physiological results of laughter. Laughter stimulates the peristaltic movement of the bowels, and massages the digestive organs. It increases respiratory activity, oxygen exchange and the heart rate. And it may even stimulate the release of endorphins (the body's natural painkillers) in the brain. Whatever the reasons, laughter remains as valuable to our health today as when the quote at the beginning of this chapter was first written down 3,000 years ago.

LAUGHTER AND STRESS

Laughter and emotional stress are not comfortable bed-fellows. In fact, it is very difficult for one to exist whilst the other is present. A good sense of humour will see you through any situation in life. One recent and very interesting study carried out at the University of Maryland concluded that laughter actually helps people solve problems and deal with stressful situations.

At the university, two groups of people were given problem solving tasks after they were shown video films. The first group were shown an educational film and the other group were shown a funny film. The group who had seen the funny film solved their tasks three times faster than the other group. A further study indicated that people who laugh have lower levels of stress hormones (adrenaline and cortisol) in their blood than people who don't laugh.

Laughter does not just help us deal with problems and situations, it helps us overcome past embarrassments, regrets and emotional hurt. How many times have you faced what seemed like a catastrophe, then a few weeks later been able to laugh about it? Didn't the laughter ease or even get rid of the hurt or embarrassment?

How much easier life might be if we could learn to see the funny side sooner rather than later. For once we take life a little less seriously, we begin to see the funny side. We all make mistakes, and we all do stupid things occasionally, but so what? If we were meant to be perfect, God would have given us wings.

I am sure that there have been days in the past few months when you may have encountered upsets and disappointments and difficult situations. So consider the following story involving the first American astronaut, John Glenn. He was all kitted up, ready to enter the rocket before an Apollo mission into space, when he was approached by a reporter. 'John, what's going to happen if, after you get up into orbit, the engines fail and you can't get back down?' To which the astronaut replied 'That would really spoil my day.' It is unlikely that many people have gone through, or will go through, such a stressful situation as John Glenn faced that day, but if you can approach life's challenges with the same sense of humour, you will find that there is nothing in this world you cannot overcome.

I therefore leave you with one suggestion that will help you tackle any situation in life, whether it be illness or adversity. Ask yourself 'What is funny about this situation?' or 'What could be funny about this situation?' Then you are much more likely to see the funny side of life.

30
THE FORESIGHT
LIFEPLAN

The foresight lifeplan is a set of simple guidelines for a healthier life, a way of living in harmony with the natural laws in order to promote an active healing force and an efficient immune system and so ensure optimum health. It contains basic guidelines for preventive health care; practices that produce health. It also points out those practices that commonly create the conditions for dis-ease and that deplete the body of energy. Remember that, according to the World Health Organisation, 85 per cent of all disease is preventable. One ounce of prevention is worth a pound of cure.

However the complete foresight lifeplan is not suitable all the time or for everybody. For instance, if you have a broken leg, you won't do it any good by exercising on it. If you have hyper-acidity in the stomach and intestines you should not be eating acid fruits (particularly citrus fruits) or nuts as these will aggravate the condition. The foresight lifeplan is merely a basic plan, and needs to be adapted in accordance with your iris analysis.

FOOD AND DIET

Do
- Eat plenty of fruits, nuts and vegetables.
- Eat plenty of raw foods. Raw foods should account for 50–75 per cent of the diet. Cooking destroys many nutrients, including enzymes and vitamins.
- Chew thoroughly. Digestion begins in the mouth.
- Eat whole unrefined foods.

- Eat when relaxed.
- Eat only when hungry and drink only when thirsty.
- Drink mineral/filtered/distilled water.

Don't
- Over-eat.
- Eat when emotionally upset, tired, or immediately after hard work.
- Eat meats of any kind.
- Eat hard cheeses.
- Cook with aluminium cookware or foil.
- Eat foods containing artificial preservatives, colourings or flavourings.
- Eat a heavy meal in the evening.

POSTURE

Do
- Sit and stand erect.
- Keep work or reading material near you instead of moving towards it.

Don't
- Do regular imbalanced movements, e.g. always holding the phone between the same shoulder and ear (this will create a structural imbalance, in this case leading to neck and shoulder problems).
- Sleep on a very soft mattress.

PHYSICAL ACTIVITY

Do
- Exercise regularly, using all parts of the body.
- Exercise in fresh air where possible in preference to an enclosed room. If you can only exercise in a room, make sure it is well ventilated by opening the windows.
- Exercise to the point of heavy breathing.
- Try to get outside every day.

Don't
- Exercise beyond the point of exhaustion/pain.
- Road run without good-quality running shoes.
- Lift weights in a gym with proper instruction.
- Remain in the direct sunlight without protection.

SLEEP

Do
- Go to bed before midnight.
- Make sure your room is well ventilated.
- Relax and meditate on comforting thoughts prior to retiring.

Don't
- Eat a large meal before retiring.

CLOTHING

Do
- Wear clothes of porous material (e.g. cotton).

Don't
- Wear tight constricting clothing.
- Wear synthetic fabrics next to the skin.

EMOTIONS

Do
- Find something to be grateful for every day.
- Feed your emotions with positive thoughts every day.
- Concentrate on the present moment.
- Pursue constructive goals.
- Engage in activities which give you fulfillment.

- Release negative emotions – fear, grief, jealousy, anger.
- Practise forgiveness – resentment is a heavy burden to carry throughout life.
- Seek the good qualities in other people rather than the bad.
- Seek the positive side in life rather than the negative/bad.
- Seek your God.

Don't
- Dwell on the past or worry about the future – concentrate on today.

31
CHOICES

I have set before you life and death, blessing and curse; therefore choose life that both you and your seed may live.

Deuteronomy 30,19

You have a choice, and you can choose now, today. The past is finished, yesterday is a memory. Tomorrow doesn't have to be like yesterday. It is only when we do the things we have always done that we get what we have always got.

The power of our lives is in the present moment. It is the choices we make today and the actions we take today that will create our tomorrow. It is sometimes difficult to accept that we have the power to shape our future; it is somehow easier to believe that someone else or something else is the cause of problems, whether it be God, the weather, the boss, the doctor, or even the naturopath. That way we can blame someone or something else and make them responsible for putting things right again.

But we all know, deep down, that the world does not work like that. The fact remains that we are in control, we are in charge, and we are responsible for the running of our lives. We are already creating our tomorrows. Each and every moment of the day we are faced with choices – what to do and what not to do, what to think and what not to think. We choose our thoughts as surely as we choose our actions. And I know of no more enlightening experience, at least in my own life, than the awareness and realisation that we choose our destiny, that we actually have a say in our lives.

For centuries we have been confused in the field of health and medicine. We have been taught that our health, or lack of it, is the wrath of God or the outcome of chance; either we have been cursed by the force that created us or we have received a poor hand in the card game of life. Only now are we beginning to understand that we always were, and always will be, in control; we are driving the vehicles we call our bodies, and we shape the vehicles of our children.

Once we realise that we are responsible for our own health, we no longer need to suffer ill-health. If there is one law operating in the universe, it is the law that we reap only that which we sow – as one writer put it, 'The game of life is a game of boomerangs'. Whatever we put out we get back, and this is the very cornerstone of preventive health care and the underlying message of iridology. Health is not the result of divine curse, or of bad luck; it is the natural outcome of our thoughts and actions.

I leave you with the ancient story of a wise old man who knew the answers to most questions asked of him. One day a young boy decided to trick him. The child caught a bird and, holding it behind his back, he took it to the old man and asked 'Old man what do I hold behind my back?' The wise old man replied, 'Why, of course, you are holding a bird behind your back.'

The boy thought that the wise old man might get the answer to his first question right, but was ready to trick him with the second question by asking whether the bird was dead or alive. If the old man said 'Alive' the boy would break the bird's neck and show it to be dead; and if the old man said 'Dead', the boy would let the bird fly away, showing it to be alive.

And so the boy asked the wise old man, 'Old man, is the bird dead or alive?', and the wise old man looked deep into the child's eyes and replied, 'My child, that life is in your hands'.

The same words ring true for us. Our health and our happiness are not determined by circumstances; they are determined by us and are therefore our responsibilities. For if you are quiet, and if you take the trouble to listen very carefully, you may hear the still small voice of the Creator answer all your anxieties; whether you are to be happy or sad, healthy or diseased, the voice answers 'It is in your hands'.

APPENDIX

HERBAL REMEDIES

How to make herbal remedies
Herbs can be made up in several ways.

- *Teas* Herbal teas are made by infusing the herbs in boiled water (one cup of water for one teaspoon of herb) which are then left for five minutes. Honey and a slice of lemon may be added to taste. Many herbal teas are an acquired taste and therefore start by making them weak by using slightly less herb leaves or root per cup.
- *Tablets* These can of course be purchased direct from a herbalist, but a cheaper way is to by the powdered herbs, combine them with a hard-set honey into a dough consistency and then roll the mixture into little balls the size of a pea. Take one or two with each meal.
- *Capsules* These again may be purchased but tend, like tablets, to be expensive. They are made up using gelatine (which is derived from dead animals).
- *Tincture* This is made by leaving the herb in alcohol spirit for several months so that the medicinal qualities may be drawn in a concentrated form into the alcohol.
- *Fluid Extracts* These are strong preparations and are purchased direct from a herbalist.

I have found that it is better to take herbal remedies for six days and then rest them for one day. I have no logical explanation for this although it is written in the Bible that everything in nature needs a period of rest: the land should be rested from cultivation for one in every seven years, whereas humans and agricultural animals are commanded to rest for one day in every seven. It may just be that the human's body healing force works best when it is given a rest from any kind of stimulant once every seven days. This may give the body a chance to recover and build without being reliant on the herb. Whatever the reason, my experience suggests that the body reacts best if for one day each week it is allowed to rest. In fact, a one day fast each week has been recommended throughout the ages by sages and healers to maintain strong health. If you are in good health and your medical practitioner agrees, try it and see.

HERBS FOR HEALTH

Listed below are some of the better known herbs which are commonly used not just to treat various ailments but also to keep the body healthy.

Aloe Vera The aloe is a cactus which is absolutely miraculous when applied externally in the treatment of all types of burns and skin irritations. Rubbed onto the skin it helps protect against sunburn.

Buchu Buchu is a diuretic and helps flush and cleanse the kidneys. It is used for all kidney and bladder infections and disorders.

Burdock Burdock is a blood purifier and like cayenne stimulates the skin to sweat and remove toxins. It is commonly used by herbalists in the treatment of all skin complaints.

Camomile Camomile is a commonly used herb taken in the form of a tea to help calm and soothe the nervous system and relieve cramps associated with the menstrual cycle.

Capsicum (Cayenne pepper) This is a wonderful herb which emanates from South America and is used extensively for minor stomach and intestinal upsets. It stimulates circulation and is excellent not only in times of crisis (e.g. colds and 'flu) but also helps to strengthen and cleanse the immune system. It is particularly noted for its ability to help produce perspiration and thus eliminate toxins through the skin.

Centaury Known on the Continent as 'a thousand medicines', centaury is a widely used herb particularly for liver and digestive complaints. It helps flush the liver and has a cleansing effect on the intestines. Only beware, this is an extremely bitter herb and is best taken in fluid extract form or alternatively as a cold tea.

Comfrey Comfrey is a great healer when applied externally to inflammations, swellings and most often to bone fractures and bruises.

Echinacea A natural blood and lymph cleanser which contains anti-bacterial qualities.

Garlic Garlic is a well-known blood cleanser having approximately one-tenth of the strength of penicillin. It helps bring down blood cholesterol levels and is used in the treatment of virtually all diseases and infections. Regular use of garlic helps keep the blood pure and free from bacterial infection.

Ginger Ginger is excellent to soothe irritations in the stomach and intestines and to stimulate circulation, particularly when applied externally. The Chinese add ginger to massage oils to relieve muscular cramps and tension and stimulate the skin, and they also add it to hot foot-baths.

Lady's slipper This is one of the strongest herbal sedatives and particularly useful for chronic nervous tension and insomnia. As a preventive measure it may be taken in the evening to help induce sleep and at times when emotional tension is building up.

Mustard Mustard is a mild laxative and blood purifier but is also excellent when the aroma is inhaled for breaking up old mucus in the lungs. Mustard gas was used in the First World War as a weapon but soldiers who were only mildly affected by it were cured of their bronchial diseases.

Sarsaparilla Another strong blood purifier and used historically in the treatment of skin complaints. It also contains hormone-like substances and has been used to help balance glandular disorders. As a preventive medicine it is an excellent spring clean herb taken for 40 days.

Slippery elm Slippery elm is the inner lining of the bark of an elm tree and used as a powder helps to absorb excess acidity and soothe inflammations. It may be taken internally for hyperacidity in the stomach and intestines and also applied externally to soothe inflamed skin irritations (e.g. eczema, psoriasis, dermatitis, etc.).

Valerian root A well-known relaxant which has a sedative and calming effect on the nervous system without causing drowsiness.

BIOCHEMIC TISSUE SALTS

The biochemic system of medicine was formulated by Dr Wilhem H. Scheussler of Oldenburg, Germany who believed that disease within the body was always associated with a deficiency of one or more inorganic substances which he called 'tissue salts'.

Biochemic tissue salts are very simply inorganic minerals that are made up homoeopathically so there is, in fact, very little mineral content in them. They do not supply the body with vast quantities of minerals but rather have the effect of enabling the body to utilise the minerals it already has. Often health problems occur *not* from lack of vitamins/minerals but from having an inability to absorb or utilise them properly. This may be due to taking synthetically prepared vitamin/mineral tablets and/or poor diet. For example, refined white flour products leach the body of vital elements including calcium and zinc because in order to convert the starch into energy, the body needs the elements which ordinarily come with the food in nature!

The 12 tissue salts

- Calcium fluoride
- Calcium phosphate
- Calcium sulphate
- Ferrum phosphate
- Potassium chloride
- Potassium phosphate
- Potassium sulphate
- Magnesium phosphate
- Sodium chloride
- Sodium phosphate
- Sodium sulphate
- Silicon dioxide

As with all homoeopathically prepared tablets, these should not be taken with food or coffee/tea. Four tablets should be taken on the tongue three times a day. Try not to touch the tablets with your hands as this may affect the remedy. Instead drop them into the lid of the container and then onto the tongue. These remedies have no known side effects and they are not habit forming.

HOT AND COLD FOOTBATHS

Hot and cold footbaths are a wonderful tonic and one of the most effective forms of hydrotherapy, used for centuries by European physicians and popularised by the famous physician Sebastian Kniepp. This simple and easy-to-perform therapy is an excellent way of helping to improve blood and lymphatic circulation throughout the body. It is used as a general tonic to help speed up recovery from illness and is particularly useful in all circulatory disorders.

All you need is two bowls, each large enough to put both feet in and deep enough to allow the water level to reach just above the ankle. One bowl should be filled with hot water (as hot as the feet can stand) into which you can add oil of ginger (something the Chinese have been doing for thousands of years for additional stimulation) and the other with cold water (again as cold as the feet can stand).

Place both feet into the hot water for three minutes followed by one minute in the cold and then repeat the process two or three times. This should be done on a daily basis if possible.

RAW FRUIT AND VEGETABLE JUICES

Raw freshly made juices are a wonderful way of cleansing the body and providing vital nutrients. The juices contain distilled water which is a solvent and therefore helps cleanse the body, and they are packed with enzymes, vitamins and minerals which are quickly and easily absorbed into the blood stream. You do not need to worry about pesticides or chemical residues, which cling to the cell walls of the vegetable or fruit and are not left in the juice itself. Raw juices have been used for centuries in nature cure clinics the world over, with great success, and are excellent in maintaining good health. However *do not* try and drink vast quantities thinking that if a little is good, a lot is better – sunshine is essential to life but too much can cause skin cancer!

All fruit juices are extremely cleansing although the high acid content in citrus fruits may irritate people with lymphatic constitutions. The following vegetable juices are nourishing and cleansing, although as with food, do not take or drink large quantities (i.e. more than two to three medium glasses per day) without supervision.

Beetroot juice Helps build up red corpuscles in the blood. It has a cleansing effect on the liver and may, if taken on its own, cause slight nausea. It is best taken with three parts carrot juice.

Cabbage juice   Extremely cleansing and helps heal acid irritations and ulcers in the stomach and intestines. However, it may cause the generation of gas as a result of putrefactive matter being broken down in the intestines by the juice.

Carrot juice   High in vitamin A as well as a host of other nutrients, carrot juice is a pleasant sweet-tasting drink that helps the body cleanse the blood, resist infection, nourish the skin and the nervous system.

Celery juice   High in magnesium and iron necessary to nourish the blood and maintain optimum fluidity of the blood. Celery juice is pleasant to take and can be mixed with carrot juice.

Cucumber juice   One of the best natural diuretics known, promoting the flow of urine. The high silica content makes it useful to strengthen hair, skin, nails and gums.

Potato juice   Raw potatoes are high in potassium which helps in cases of excess acidity in the body.

Spinach juice   Raw spinach helps cleanse and tone the entire intestinal tract. (However, if the spinach is cooked its oxalic acid content will often crystallise in the kidneys.)

Tomato juice   Rich in sodium, calcium, potassium and magnesium, tomato juice is nutritious and cleansing. (Again, the oxalic acids crystallise in the kidney and bladder if the tomatoes are cooked.)

SKIN BRUSHING

Brushing the skin with a hard-bristled brush helps to stimulate blood and lymph circulation, promotes the elimination of toxins through the skin, and removes old skin cells which often clog the pores in the skin. It is done by simply using a natural fibre skin brush and making firm brush strokes always in the direction of the heart to encourage the flow of blood back towards the heart (i.e. up the legs, up the arms, up the abdomen, down the neck and inwards across the chest and shoulder blades). Seven brush strokes over each area is sufficient when done on a daily basis. However do not do this more regularly than once a day or it may induce constipation due to excessive wastes being eliminated. Do not brush too hard to begin with if you have a sensitive skin.

THE ANTI-ACID DIET

The anti-acid diet is designed for those people prone to, or suffering from, hyper-acidity in the body, particularly in the stomach and intestines. People with an acid constitution need to be particularly careful to maintain a balance of acid/alkaline-forming foods in order to avoid a build up of excess acidity in the body.

The body's chemistry is 20 per cent acid and 80 per cent alkaline. Therefore to retain the right chemical balance, our diet should be made up of 20 per cent acid-forming foods, and 80 per cent alkaline-forming foods.

The main acid-forming foods
- Meats, poultry and fish.
- All dairy produce, save natural yoghurt.
- White flour and white sugar products.
- Wheat (this also contains high amounts of gluten, a sticky protein substance that, taken in excess, irritates the walls of the small intestine.)
- Cooked tomatoes and cooked spinach – high in oxalic acid, which crystallises in the kidneys.
- Vinegars (except cider vinegar, which is alkaline).
- Acid fruits – citrus fruits (oranges, grapefruits, lemon and pineapple), as well as strawberries and rhubarb.

- Nuts (except almonds and hazelnuts).
- Tea, coffee and alcohol.

The main alkaline-forming foods
- Fresh fruits and vegetables, except those mentioned above. (Fruits and vegetables should not be mixed at the same meal as the acids are not compatible in the digestive process.)
- Barley, millet, buckwheat and rice – all excellent for soothing the intestinal tract. Buckwheat and millet are both highly alkaline, whereas wholegrain rice and barley are neutral but soothe the intestinal tract with their soft fibre content.
- Dried figs are highly alkaline.
- Almonds and hazelnuts.
- Herbal teas.
- Slippery elm – this is really a wonderful food, which absorbs excess acid, not just in the intestines, but from all soft tissues in the body, and helps eliminate the acids from the system. A sufficient dose is one teaspoon mixed with muesli or hot cereal or taken in tablet form.
- Fresh fruit and vegetable juices, especially cabbage and potato, have a powerful alkalising effect on the blood.

The emotions
Please remember that it is not foods alone that cause acidity. One can eat the best foods in the world and still create acidity through negative emotions (e.g. anger, resentment, jealousy, etc.). The mind is more powerful than we realise, and mental and spiritual attitudes are vital in maintaining health.

GLOSSARY

Acute A condition arising suddenly and manifesting intense severity, usually accompanied by pain and inflammation, but lasting only a short time.

Adhesions Tissues in the body stuck together.

Alimentary tract Gastro-intestinal tract – the gut.

Arcus senilis A white/yellow arc around the periphery of the upper section of the iris which often leads to the formation of a cholesterol ring.

Ascending colon The section of large intestine on the right side of the body rising from the appendix to the liver.

Autonomic nerve wreath (ANW) The wreath seen around the pupil usually situated approximately a third of the distance between the pupil and outer edge of the iris. It indicates the condition of the autonomic nervous system and also the shape of the large and small intestines.

Cataract A disease of the eye in which the crystalline lens of the eye becomes partially or totally opaque.

Cholesterol ring (also called sodium or mineral ring) A white, or yellowish-white ring around outer edge of the iris indicating hardening of the arteries (arteriosclerosis) caused by excess sodium/calcium deposits and high levels of cholesterol.

Chronic Long-standing condition seen as a dark discoloration in iris.

Closed lacuna A lacuna with both ends closed, indicating an area of the body that is not receiving sufficient nutrients or that is unable to eliminate toxins efficiently.

Colitis Inflammation of the colon.

Colon Term for the large intestine (ascending, transverse and descending).

Congenital A condition existing from birth, although not necessarily hereditary.

Constitution The physical and psychological make-up of a person, revealing that person's general state of health and inherent strengths and weaknesses.

Defects   Small lacunae which appear in a variety of shapes (e.g. lancet, pear, asparagus, diamond, etc.). A serious condition which needs prompt attention.

Degenerative stage   The final stage of degeneration and tissue breakdown, seen in the iris as black discolorations.

Descending colon   The section of the large intestine on left side of body going down from the spleen to the rectum.

Eliminative channels   Five main channels for elimination of toxic waste from the body are lungs, bowels, kidneys, skin and lymph.

Glaucoma   A disease of the eye in which excessive pressure within the eyeball causes damage to the optic disc, leading to impaired vision, sometimes progressing to blindness.

Healing crisis   A recurrence of previously experienced symptoms caused by the body eliminating toxins.

Hering's Law of Cure   Healing proceeds from within out, from the top down, in reverse order and from vital organs to less vital organs.

Hyperacid stomach   Excess HC1 (hydrochloric) acid in the stomach zone seen as a bright white discoloration (acute) or a white/silver halo (sub-chronic) in the stomach ring in the iris.

Hypo-acidity   Lack of acid and diminished function.

Impactions   Bowel pockets formed by gas pressure, or feces impacted onto the colon wall retaining putrefactive matter which is not eliminated in daily bowel movements.

Inflammation   The reaction of body tissue to injury or infection characterised by heat, redness, swelling and pain.

Iris   The coloured muscular diaphragm in the eye that surrounds and controls the size of the pupil, and reflects and affects the tissues throughout the body.

Lacuna(e)   A 'hole' seen in the iris fibres which may appear in a variety of shapes and sizes, and indicates inherent weakness in the tissue.

Lymphatic rosary   A string of small puffy clouds in

the lymphatic zone of the iris that range in colour from white to yellow or brown and indicates congestion of the lymphatic system and an excess of mucus.

Metabolism The conversion of foodstuffs into energy.

Naturopathy System of remedial treatment based upon the vital healing force within nature and within humans, which seeks to support and strengthen that force by natural means.

Nerve rings Also referred to as cramp rings and tension rings seen as circular contractions of iris fibres and indicating the accumulation of physiological and emotional stress and tension.

Open lacunae Lacunae beginning toward ANW and opening outwards. They indicate that whilst the organ is weak, it is still receiving adequate nutrients and is able to eliminate metabolic wastes.

Psoric spots Pigmentation lying above the iris structure which indicates accumulation of chemicals and metabolic wastes.

Pterygium Yellow thickened membranous tissue seen in the sclera which also may cover part of the iris, affecting those areas.

Pupil The dark circular aperture at the centre of the iris through which light enters the inner eye.

Radii solaris Spikes emanating from the intestinal zone (caused by impactions) and the ANW indicating a possible reflex disturbance to the area of the body to which the spikes are pointing.

Reflex A specific and foreseeable response to a given stimulus.

Retina The light-sensitive membrane forming the inner lining of the posterior wall of the eyeball composed largely of specialised terminal expansion of the optic nerve.

Sclera The white of eye surrounding the iris.

Scurf rim A darkening in the skin zone of the iris due to the retention of wastes, suppression and inactivity of the skin.

Skin zone The most outward zone on iris.

Stomach halo A circular white/silver halo in the stomach zone around the pupil.

Tophi (tophus) Discolorations in the iris resembling flakes, clouds or spots that range from white to yellow in colour and indicate congestion.

Toxins Pollutants, body wastes, minerals, drugs and chemicals which collect in the blood and lymph and put a stress on all the eliminative channels of the body.

Transverse colon The section of the colon which goes across the upper abdomen between the liver on the right-hand side and the spleen on the left.

Transversals White or vascularised acute signs which run across the normal fibre direction, indicating adhesions, and acute to chronic irritability.

USEFUL
ADDRESSES

The following organisations run courses and seminars on Iridology as well as providing a list of practitioners:

USA

National Iridology Research Association
PO Box 33637
Seattle
WA 98133

Dr Bernard Jensen
Hidden Valley Health Ranch
Route 1
Box 52
Escondido
CA 92025

Center for Effective Living
450 W. Hillsboro Boulevard
Deerfield Beach
FL 33441

CANADA

The Canadian Institute of Iridology
Suite 201
2500 Bathurst St
Toronto M6B 2Y8

BIBLIOGRAPHY

Dr H.W. Anderschou, *Iris Science*, Published by Dr H.W. Anderschou, 1916 (out of print)

H. Benjamin, *Better Sight Without Glasses*, Health for all Publishing Co., 1929

Norman Cousins, *Anatomy of an Illness*, Bantam Books, 1979

Peter Cox, *Why You Don't Need Meat*, Thorsons, 1986

P. Cox and P. Brusseau, *The Quick Cholesterol Clean-out*, Century Hutchinson, 1989

Viktor Frankl, *Man's Search for Meaning*, Washington Square Press, 1985

Dr R. Gray, *The Colon Health Handbook*, Rockbridge Publishing Co., 1980

Dorothy Hall, *Iridology*, Angus & Robertson, 1980

Aldous Huxley, *The Art of Seeing*, Triad Grafton, 1985

Ivan Illich, *Limits to Medicine: Medical Nemesis*, Pelican, 1977

Dr Bernard Jensen, *The Science and Practice of Iridology*, published by B Jensen, 1952

T. Kriege, *Fundamental Basis of Irisdiagnosis*, L.N. Fowler & Co. Ltd., 1975

T. Kriege and A.W. Priest, *Disease Signs in the Iris*, L.N. Fowler & Co. Ltd., 1985

Dr Colin B. Lessell, *The Biochemic Handbook*, Thorsons, 1984

Henry Lindlahr MD., *Iris diagnosis and other diagnostic methods*, The C.W. Daniel Co Ltd. 1985

Wataru Ohashi, *Do-it-yourself Shiatsu* Unwin Paperbacks, 1977

Anthony Robbins, *Unlimited Power*, Simon & Schuster Ltd., 1986

Florence Scovel-Shinn, *The Game of Life and How to Play it*, L.N. Fowler & Co. Ltd., 1925

Dr B.S. Siegel, *Love, Medicine, and Miracles*, Arrow, 1986

N.W. Walker D.Sci. *Raw Vegetable Juices*, Jove Publications, 1970

Antoine de Saint-Exupéry, *The Little Prince*, William Heinemann Ltd., 1945

Doris Grant and Jean Joice, *Food Combining for Health*, Thorsons, 1984

INDEX

Page numbers in *italic* refer to the illustrations